OPEN
SIDE

OPEN
SIDE

SAM WARBURTON

WITH BORIS STARLING

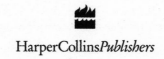

HarperCollins*Publishers*

HarperCollins*Publishers*
1 London Bridge Street
London SE1 9GF

www.harpercollins.co.uk

First published by HarperCollins*Publishers* 2019

3 5 7 9 10 8 6 4

© Sam Warburton 2019

Sam Warburton asserts the moral right to
be identified as the author of this work

Extract on page 105 from *Western Mail*, 17 October, 2011
courtesy of *Western Mail*/Media Wales

A catalogue record of this book is
available from the British Library

HB ISBN 978-0-00-833657-8
PB ISBN 978-0-00-833658-5

Printed and bound in Great Britain by
CPI Group (UK) Ltd, Croydon

MIX
Paper from
responsible sources
FSC
www.fsc.org
FSC™ C007454

This book is produced from independently certified FSC™ paper
to ensure responsible forest management.

For more information visit: www.harpercollins.co.uk/green

To my wife Rachel, daughter Anna, my family
and close friends – thanks for being on the journey
with me, supporting me and helping me through all
the tough times. I could never have done
it without you.

CONTENTS

CONTENTS

PROLOGUE

Friday, 30 June 2017
The Rydges Hotel, Wellington, New Zealand

Two in the morning.

Can't sleep. The witching hour, when the darkness comes flooding in: thoughts tumbling and cascading over each other like a Snowdonia river in full spate. The darkness comes flooding in, and it's all I can do to stop it drowning me.

Everything hurts. My body, my mind, my heart. Everything. I'm a wreck.

It's easier to list the parts of me that aren't in pain. My eyelashes. That's pretty much it. I've had more than 20 injuries over my career: the concussions, the broken jaw, the plate in my eye socket, the trapped shoulder nerve, the hamstring torn clean off the bone, the knee ligaments.

Before I go out to play these days, I have to neck painkillers while the physios strap me up like an Egyptian mummy. I have to stand there butt naked in front of them, cupping my twig and berries, while they bind my knees, my ankles, my shoulders and my elbows.

It's not just tonight. It's the relentless grind: week on week, month on month, year on year. Smash and be smashed. Try to recover. Smash and be smashed again. The equivalent of strapping myself into a car like a crash test dummy and driving it at a wall every weekend.

I get out of bed. Shards of pain as my feet touch the floor. I push myself slowly upright, gritting my teeth as the aches flare and settle.

If my body's only at around 70 per cent fitness, my mind feels around half that. I'm exhausted, but also wired: antsy, yet craving rest. Yes, these are the small hours when everything seems worse, but even in broad daylight the doubts and questions are never far away.

Sam Warburton shouldn't be captain.

Sam Warburton shouldn't be playing.

Sam Warburton's past it.

What I know is that there are plenty of people out there who think that.

What I fear is that they might be right.

I take one step, gingerly, then another, and another. Walking – hobbling, more like – across the carpet over to the window. I pull back the curtains and look out.

Below me is the Wellington waterfront. It's quiet and empty now, but earlier this evening it was packed, as it will be later tonight and tomorrow night. Many of these people will be wearing red rugby shirts and will have saved up for years to come all the way across the world just to watch us play.

Because tomorrow evening I'm going to lead out the British and Irish Lions for the second of three Tests against the All Blacks. We lost the first in Auckland last week, which means we have to win this one to stay in the series. I've played in some big games in my life – World Cup semi-finals, Grand Slam deciders, Lions Tests against Australia – but nothing that comes close to this.

Nothing that comes remotely close.

The best of the Home Nations, a once-every-four-years touring team, against the double world champions. I came off the bench in Auckland, but now I'm starting and I simply have to deliver.

It should be the highlight of my career. It feels like anything but.

This is a game that's been the biggest part of my life for almost two decades, a game that has largely defined me. It's a game I love. Rather, it's a game I thought I loved. Right now, I hate it.

I want to be one of those fans, on the piss and singing their hearts out, with no problem more pressing than who gets the next round in. Instead, I'm here, torturing myself with questions to which I have no answer. *Why? Why am I doing this to myself? Why am I putting myself through all this pain, all this pressure, when I could be doing something – anything – else? Why am I in a job which right now I detest?*

Round and round and round. Body, mind and heart. Physical stress, mental stress and emotional stress, all working on and off each other. I feel as though I'm in a submarine going deeper and deeper, springing leaks as the hull creaks and flexes, and soon I'll come to the point of no return, the moment when the pressure gets too much and crushes me like a tin can.

Two in the morning, and no one to talk to.

For once in my career I've chosen to have a room on my own rather than share with a team-mate. It's the captain's prerogative, to have a room to himself, but one I've rarely used as I don't like to be set apart from the other boys.

This time, I have. I've told everyone it's because I need the sleep, which is true – my daughter Anna's not far off a year old, and like all babies she's up more times in the night than a vampire – but it's not the whole truth either.

It's because I need the space too. The six weeks of this tour are what my entire career has been building towards, and I want to win so much, *so much*, that the desire is almost in itself a physical pain. *Another* physical pain, more like.

A submarine. A volcano. All this pain bubbling up inside me, and if I don't deal with it, it's going to explode and consume me in all its molten fury.

I need to talk to someone. There are several people I could call, but there's only one person I know will really understand. I dial her number.

'Sam?' Her voice is full of concern. It's lunchtime back home in Cardiff. She knows what time it is where I am, and that I wouldn't be phoning for no reason.

'I've had enough, Mum.' My throat is tight with the effort of not bursting into tears. 'I really have. I'm just going to go.'

'Go where?'

'To the airport. Do a bunk. Leave all my kit here, get on the first plane home. I'll be in the air before they realise I've gone.'

* * *

4

I didn't, of course. Can you imagine the headlines?

LIONS CAPTAIN DOES MIDNIGHT FLIT.

WARBURTON QUITS.

THE RUNAWAY SKIPPER.

I'd never have lived it down, and rightly so.

But at the time I was deadly serious. And no one knew, apart from my mum. She talked me down: told me that I didn't owe anything to anyone, so all I had to do was get through this week and the next and then the series would be over and I could do what I wanted.

She was right, of course. She knew the way love for and hatred of rugby oscillated within me, because they did for her too. She loved what the game had given me and the pleasure I'd got from it, but she hated seeing me beaten up, or under the knife, or criticised. Even though I was 6 ft 2 and 16 stone, I was still her little boy.

No one knew, apart from my mum. The spectators in the Westpac Stadium the following evening certainly didn't know when they watched one of the most titanic and dramatic Test matches imaginable. And there's no reason they should have known. The rugby public see what the players want them to see, and no more.

I played most of my career with 7 on my back. For me 7 has, in rugby terms, always been a sacred number. This book is arranged according to that number. There are seven main chapters, each centred on a different rugby ground in which something important in my life happened: a red card or two, a debut, a barnstorming run, a horrific injury, a goal-line stand, a split-second decision with a referee.

In between those chapters are seven sections centred around

different aspects of leadership (Personality, Professionalism, Performance, Perspective, Positivity, Persistence and People), because over the years as captain for Wales and the Lions I've learned a bit about all of those too.

Number 7 is the openside flanker, the one who packs down in a scrum furthest from the near touchline and therefore has more of the field to patrol than number 6, the blindside. I've played a bit at six too, and in writing this I realised that openside and blindside aren't just positions on the pitch. They're also reflections of how much people really know about the life of a professional rugby player.

Most of the time, that knowledge is the blindside, the narrow side. You see us on match day, and maybe in social media videos or promotional appearances too. That's some of our life, but it's only a very, very small part. The rest of it, those wide expanses which the number 7 needs to patrol, is kept hidden.

This is the story of those expanses, the parts of the iceberg beneath the surface. It's a story of highs and lows, of triumph and disaster. It's a story of what it's really like to be in the thick of it, on and off the pitch. It's not every rugby player's story, but it's my story, told as clearly and honestly as I can.

This is my open side.

1

WHITCHURCH

51.5132°N, 3.2234°W

2002

We're playing Llanhari. Their number 8's a big lad, running to fat, and he's nasty too. We're not yet a quarter of the way through the match when I see him choking our scrum-half: proper choking, lifting him off his feet while holding him by the neck, all that.

I see red. I smash into this lad as hard as I can, picking him up and throwing him down, head first. I don't know how dangerous this is, of course; none of us do. I'm just enraged that he's picking on one of my team-mates, and the smallest lad on the pitch to boot. Besides, dump tackling's my trademark, my way of stamping my authority on the game and getting my team behind me. In each game I play, I don't look to dump the smallest guy on their team, but the biggest one.

Having seen red once, I see it again when the ref sends me off. I can't complain, but equally I won't apologise. I'm not a dirty player, and I never do anything illegal unless provoked; but if someone starts something, I'm determined to be the one to finish it. And I'll never back down from defend-ing a team-mate. Even a chopsing scrum-half, talking back to people.

1995. 'I want to be a footballer.'

I'm seven years old. Mum's putting me and my twin brother Ben to bed. We've been playing football all afternoon, like we always do. There's a grass verge on the corner of our street, and we play there for hours at a time. The neighbours must hate us, but we don't know, and even if we did we wouldn't care. We're just kids playing football.

When he's not on shift at Whitchurch fire station, Dad plays with us. He was pretty good when he was younger – he had a sweet left foot and a trial for Bristol Rovers – but he couldn't be bothered with the whole professional lifestyle, certainly not in the days before the big money came flooding in. He just wanted to play locally. Now he teaches us how to pass, and control, and shoot, and head the ball: all the things that will make us better players.

We've both got little Spurs kits. Mine has 'Sam, 9' on the back; Ben's has 'Ben, 10.' Dad's been a Spurs fan all his life; he was born in the northwest London suburb of Kingsbury, even though his family are originally from Bury, and he came to Cardiff via Birmingham. 'Once Tottenham, always Tottenham,' he says. Playing for Spurs and Wales, that's my dream.

'Really?' Mum says. 'You want to be a footballer?'

She had Ben and me five weeks premature. One of the mater-nity nurses at Heath Hospital took one look at how small we were and said the words no self-respecting Welsh person ever wants to hear. Mum and Dad have, laughing, told us often enough what those words were.

'Well,' I reply, mimicking what the maternity nurse said, 'I'm never going to be a rugby player, am I?'

Ben and I are playing with our toys on the floor. Our favourites are Action Man (obviously) and Biker Mice from Mars. We take their clothes off and play with them. When Dad finds them naked, he puts their clothes back on. We take their clothes off again when we next play with them.

'Carolyn,' Dad says to Mum. 'I think the boys might be gay.'

Actually, we're just transfixed by the muscle definition on Action Man and the Biker Mice.

1997. Ben and I play centre-back for Llanishen Fach Primary School. We're as good as most kids our age, but now and then we come up against someone special. And there's no one more special than this kid who plays for Eglwys Newydd. We know he must be good even before the match begins, because he's wearing adidas Predators.

He's got everything: ridiculous levels of skill, pace to burn and stamina that means he can keep going all match. When he dribbles, it's like the ball is stuck to his laces. He's so good that we need half a team to stop him, and even if we do manage that it just means we've had to leave two or three of his team-mates unmarked.

He might be only nine years old, but news of his talent has spread far and wide. We hear parents whispering to each other on the touchline. *Did you see him play at that tournament in*

Newport? There were some pro scouts there, you know. Southampton have signed him to their academy.

Look on the bright side, Ben and I tell each other. When we go to Whitchurch in a couple of years, he'll be on our side rather than against us.

We ask what his name is.

He's called Gareth Bale.

There's a special needs section at school, for kids with learning difficulties and the like. One of these kids latches onto me a bit and follows me into my lessons even though it makes him late for his own. Some of my mates laugh at him and tell him to get lost, but I always try and make time for him.

We're playing cricket in the yard, and this same kid is there. He's batting and he's not very good. He swipes at the ball, missing it by a mile. The lad playing wicketkeeper catches it and throws the ball in the air. 'You're out,' he says.

'No,' I say. 'He's not.'

'He is.'

'He was nowhere near it, and you know it.'

'He hit it.'

'You only want him out so someone else can have a go.'

'Well, he's rubbish, isn't he?'

'If you want him out, then you get him out.'

'He *is* out.'

The argument turns into a scrap, and it only ends when the headmistress comes to break us up. In her office, she asks me what happened, and I tell her the truth. This kid was being bullied, and I hate bullies. I don't even know where that comes from, just that I do. I can't stand bullying, and I won't stand by when it happens and can do something about it.

1998. Ten years old, Llanishen Fach. We're playing touch rugby: Bluebirds v Blackbirds. The Bluebirds are the rugby boys, even though they've named their team after Cardiff City football club; the Blackbirds are the footballers (or, as the rugby boys like to call them, the losers). I'm playing for the Blackbirds. I've never played rugby, no one in our family's ever played, I don't like the look of it, and a game of touch doesn't make me change my mind. It's a rubbish game. You can't pass it forwards, you can't tackle people, you can't kick it.

I must have changed at least one of the teacher's minds, though, as I'm picked to play in the next rugby match. Full contact, not touch. They want me to play on the wing, as I'm quick: when it comes to sports-day sprints, I'm either winning them or pretty close.

I don't want to play. I *really* don't want to.

Match day comes. I'm terrified. I go from lesson to lesson, wondering how I can pretend to be injured, or hoping that the match will be called off. The clock ticks round. We're due to play after the school day's ended, so when the bell goes and all the kids who aren't playing go home as usual, that's just what I do. Sneak out, follow them through the gates and leg it home.

'I thought you had a match,' Dad says over tea.

'Got cancelled,' I reply, quite a lot more coolly than I feel.

Next day at school, no one says anything. All morning I'm waiting for one of the teachers to ask where I was, but they don't. By lunchtime I'm beginning to think I've got away with it. I'm in the yard with my mates, playing around, when I sense more than see the other kids stop what they're doing.

I turn around. The headmaster, Frank Rees, is coming towards me. The whole place is still; there's not a kid born who'd want to miss one of their fellow pupils being reamed out in front of the whole school. It's the kind of thing they'll be talking about for weeks afterwards. They all back away a little, as if the trouble I'm clearly in is going to be somehow contagious, but they make sure to stay well within earshot.

'Where were you yesterday afternoon?' Mr Rees asks.

It doesn't really matter what excuse I give, as he knows it's going to be a lie. He gives me a bollocking: not a shouting or screaming one, as he's not that kind of man, but stern and strict, nonetheless. If you're picked, he says, you play. It's not up to you to decide whether or not you want to.

He's right, of course, and I deserve it. By the time I get home that afternoon, he's already spoken to my parents. They tell me the same thing: don't ever bunk off again.

By the end of the year I'm playing for East Wales.

'That's why I picked you,' Mr Rees says. 'I knew how good you could be.'

1999. Being good at rugby isn't yet enough for me. I don't love it, not in the way I love football.

Cardiff Schools trial. I'm so nervous that I'm crying in the car. Just relax, Dad says, you'll be fine. But I'm not. I don't want this pressure. School matches are one thing, but this is a step up. I play badly, and not by accident. I do it on purpose, so I won't get picked for Cardiff Schools.

It works. I don't get picked. I'm glad.

Two weeks later, I'm playing for the school against Willowsbrook. No one's watching, so I don't have to throttle back or sabotage myself. I score four tries.

One of the Willowsbrook fathers comes over to Dad afterwards.

'I'm a selector for Cardiff Schools,' he says. 'Why couldn't your boy have played like that at the trial?'

2000. I'm at secondary school in Whitchurch, a school so massive (more than 2,000 kids) that they basically have to split it in two. With the move comes a jump in rugby too, from ten-a-side to the full 15.

Cardiff Schools, away to Bridgend. My first time on a bus with a bunch of strangers. I don't say much. I'm quiet, shy, watchful; not one of the inner circle who colonise the back row of the bus as though by right.

The coach tells me to stand on the sidelines. I'm not sure if I'm playing or if I'm a sub. Bridgend ship it out to their winger. He comes haring down the touchline towards me. What am I supposed to do?

Best take no chances, I reckon. I fly onto the pitch and smash him into next week. I'm still on the ground when I hear their players' disbelieving protests, and a fair bit of verbals too.

'Bloody hell,' says our coach. 'You're on the bench, you muppet.'

I come on in the second half. The Bridgend winger gives me a wide berth when I do.

* * *

We reach the semi-finals of the Welsh Cup. Playing against Pontypool, I put one of their boys into touch, and as I'm getting up I hear one of the coaches whistle softly and say, 'I've never seen an Under-12 hit so hard.'

They put me at openside, number 7, and instantly I fall in love with the position. A lot of the good kids play 7, so that's a compliment in itself, but it's more what the position demands. Sevens aren't as quick as the wingers, as strong as the props or as skilful as the fly-half, but they do have to be reasonably quick and strong and skilful: good all-rounders, the decathletes of a rugby team.

And they're always involved, which I absolutely love. I don't play rugby either to stand shivering near the touchline or to have my head up a prop's arse for 80 minutes. I want to be where the action is. When you're a 7 and doing your job properly, the ball's never far away, whether you're running support lines for your team-mates or tackling the oppo.

And tackling, as the coach on the sidelines saw, is very much my thing.

The one constant through changing teams and changing years: Ben. On that grass verge near our house or on a pitch a few minutes away, we're always playing; not just football now, but rugby and cricket too. God knows how much we cost Mum and Dad in broken windows, though of course we don't really realise that things cost money.

The other thing we don't realise is how much time we're putting in to making ourselves better, because it never seems like a chore. In years to come Malcolm Gladwell will write in his book *Outliers* that it takes 10,000 hours to really master something, and Ben and I are putting in a lot of these hours without even realising it.

We do lots of one on ones, trying to beat each other. Ben's where I get my competitive edge from. But no matter how much we want to beat each other, we always help each other along too. We make suggestions and point out where we think the other one's going wrong. We work together and look out for each other. We don't lay into each other or put each other down. We're best mates.

2001. I'm still playing football, not just for Whitchurch – such a relief to watch Gareth tormenting other defenders week in, week out, shielding the ball from three players at once and then weaving through them like a magician – but also for Lisvane. It's quite an affluent area of Cardiff, and a lot of the teams we play against take the mickey out of us for being posh lads and that. But we're good – we go a couple of years undefeated – and we can look after ourselves.

When we play Grangetown, which is a rough and tough area, I'm determined to show we're not going to let ourselves be intimidated. I come in hard on this kid, and he jumps on my back and tries to punch me. I hold his arms out like a crucifix and walk him all the way over to the ref so he can deal with him.

'You ever come past JD Sports,' this kid says afterwards, 'we'll be waiting.'

I know that he and his mates hang around there, and that a handful of them against one of me is going to be a different story. I give JD Sports a miss for the next couple of months.

Besides, I've slightly tarnished Lisvane's reputation. Before I started playing for them, they prided themselves on a spotless disciplinary record. The first season I'm there, I get two red cards and three yellows. I'm being physical rather than dirty, but it doesn't matter.

I realise that football doesn't have enough aggro for me. Football's a contact sport, but rugby's a collision sport. I need to smash people when I play.

2002. We're playing Llanhari. Their number 8's a big lad, running to fat, and he's nasty too. We're not yet a quarter of the way through the match when I see him choking our scrum-half: proper choking, lifting him off his feet while holding him by the neck, all that.

I see red. I smash into this lad as hard as I can, picking him up and throwing him down head first. I don't know how dangerous this is, of course; none of us do. I'm just enraged that he's picking on one of my team-mates, and the smallest lad on the pitch to boot. Besides, dump tackling's my trademark, my way of stamping my authority on the game and getting my team behind me. In each game I play, I don't look to dump the smallest guy on their team, but the biggest one.

Having seen red once, I see it again when the ref sends me off. I can't complain, but equally I won't apologise. I'm not a dirty player, and I never do anything illegal unless provoked; but if someone starts something, I'm determined to be the one to finish it. And I'll never back down from defending a team-mate. Even a chopsing scrum-half, talking back to people.

I'm waiting for the bell to start school when I first see him. He's walking across the yard with a file in his hand, and it's the way he's walking which really catches my eye: upright, purposeful, military. Even before we've exchanged a word, I know this is not a man who's going to settle for second best.

He's called Gwyn Morris, and he's our new PE teacher.

The hardest-working player will win, that's what he tells us. If you work harder than your opposition, you will win. Twice a week he has us training for an hour before school and an hour afterwards. It's not all physical stuff – we're 14 years old, and you can't push growing bodies too hard – but tactical and mental too. Mr Morris doesn't just want us to work hard, but also work smart.

Be professional, he says. Professional isn't about getting paid. It's about the way you approach things and the standards you set. It's about never being satisfied with your performance and always wanting to analyse your game, to see what you could do better next time round.

April 2003. We win the Welsh Schools championship. The final is at the Millennium Stadium, where only a few weeks earlier Wales were playing Six Nations matches against England and Ireland. (They lost both of those, and their three away matches too, for a whitewash and a wooden spoon.)

The stadium's almost empty, but it doesn't matter. Ben and I become the first twins to play at the Millennium (he plays in the centre), and I score two tries. It's a great team full of great lads. Afterwards, on the bus back to school, I have a profound sense of satisfaction: a glow, really. We did it. We worked hard for it, and we worked smart for it, and we did it.

We're singing and laughing and joking, and we feel like kings of the world.

* * *

I go for a trial at Cardiff City FC. Very quickly, I realise two things. First, there's no one here who's remotely as good as Gareth. It's hard to know quite how good someone is when you only have the schools you play by way of comparison, but Cardiff are a decent club – they'll get promotion to Division One, a step down from the Premier League, next season – so if Gareth's better than all these kids then he really must be something special.

And second, I'm not good enough. This is a step too far for me. I'm a little sad, because football's been my first love for as long as I can remember, but sooner or later I'd have to choose between football and rugby. This has made my decision for me, and deep down it's probably the decision I wanted to make anyway.

October. For our 15th birthday, Mum and Dad give Ben and me a multigym, which we put in the garage. We train there after school.

I keep thinking of what Mr Morris said. Whoever works hardest will win.

I go to the school gym at lunchtime to do weights. Sad Lad, a couple of girls call me when they see me coming out dripping with sweat. I don't care. I'm not too cool to make it look like it's all beneath me. Gym, weights, speed stuff, I'm mad for it all. I drop honey sandwiches for tins of tuna, crisps for pieces of fruit.

Whoever works hardest will win.

December. We get 21 days' holiday over Christmas, and I train at the school on 20 of those days. The 21st is Christmas Day, and the only reason I don't train then is that the place is locked and I can't get in.

Whoever works hardest will win.

2004. I start to train my mind as well as my body.

Whenever we play a match, I have to be better than my opposite number. You hear whispers on the circuit: oh, Pembrokeshire have got a good number 7, or Llanelli, or Pontypridd. And I'm thinking, *Well, he can't be as good as me. He can't be as good an athlete as me, or train as hard as me, or want it as much as I do. So no matter how good he thinks he is, I'm better.*

Whoever I play for, there's only one number 7 shirt. I'm the best 7 at Whitchurch, which is a huge school. I'm better than everyone I play against, every 7 in all 26 of Cardiff's secondary schools, and all across Wales. I'm the best 7 in Wales.

And if that's the case, and it is, then why shouldn't I be better than every schoolboy 7 in England, Scotland and Ireland, because I train harder than they do too?

I take it further. I keep hearing about this team, this almost mythical band of brothers who comprise the four Home Nations and only come together once every four years. The Lions. The British and Irish Lions.

If I'm the best schoolboy 7 among the four Home Nations, and if I keep that going into senior level, and if I'm better than everyone in a 10-year age range too – if I continue to be better than every 7 I play against, no matter how old they are – then why shouldn't I play for the Lions one day?

* * *

There's a questionnaire for the rugby team. One of the questions is 'What's your ultimate ambition?'

'British and Irish rugby legend,' I write.

'That's a bit big-headed,' says Dad when he sees it.

I shrug. 'It's true, though.'

Mr Morris nods when I tell him what I wrote. 'Aim for the stars, lad,' he says. 'If you fail, you'll still reach the sky.'

I win player of the year for Cardiff Schools Under-15s. I smile sweetly when I go up to accept the award and shake the hand of the guy presenting me with the award, but inside I'm seething.

Sure, I've won it this year, but the previous year I was on the bench all season and only played 17 minutes. I'd been a regular starter for the three years before that, and I was playing as well as anyone for Whitchurch, so why the difference?

Because the coach was getting free golf lessons off the number 7's dad, that's why.

To start with, I know her only as the badminton girl.

I hardly ever see her around. The school's so huge – 12 classes in each year – that it's split across two sites, and she's usually on the other site from me. All I know is that she plays badminton at age group for Wales, and she looks really nice.

In year 10 we get to be in a maths class together. Friday afternoon, really bored, I'm sitting with my mates at the back, and we do what boys have done in mixed classes since pretty much the dawn of time: we start rating the girls out of ten. When it comes to Rachel Thomas, I go, 'Oh, four,' just so no one thinks I'm too keen. But inside I'm thinking, *She looks*

20

really nice. Not just attractive, though of course she is – brown hair, big eyes, wide smile – but a really nice person too.

One of my mates adds her to my list on MSN Messenger, and we start chatting. Two years of messaging before we meet in person! Even though – and this is the really insane bit – all the time she lives four doors down from me, and neither of us ever know. We don't even bump into each other on the street when going to and from school. She tells me all about her family, which is tight and close like mine: she has two sisters, her parents are always loving and loyal, they've got the same values I've been brought up with.

And just as I've never had a girlfriend, she's never had a boyfriend. I ask her if we can meet up – anywhere you like, I say, even if it's just for five minutes outside your house with a bag of sweets. She's wary. She knows I play rugby, and she knows what kind of reputation the rugby boys have – girls and drinking and bad behaviour. I'm not like that, I say, but of course that's just the kind of thing someone who *was* like that would say. No point in saying it. I have to show her. Once she gets to know me, she'll see I'm really not like all the other rugby guys.

Christmas. The Lions are due to tour New Zealand next year. My folks give me a Lions jersey with 7 on the back: a real 7, with the Lions logo at the bottom. I wear this shirt everywhere, absolutely everywhere. I wear it to the gym, and out running, and in the school library when it's a non-uniform day, and when sitting at home. Sometimes I even let Mum wash it.

2005. Rugby players have a bit of an image as thick louts, and I'm determined to be neither. I'm in the top third of my classes; not super-intelligent by any means, but better than average. Only two teachers reckon I won't do well in my GCSEs. My biology teacher predicts a D, my RE teacher says E. No way, I tell them both. I'll get an A. I might not be able to work everything out for myself from scratch, but I'm good at parrot learning, and if that's what it takes then that's what it takes. You can argue that the exam system is wrong and that it doesn't take into account things that it should do, but it's like wanting to play rugby at 7 – don't bitch about it, just get on with it.

Prove the doubters wrong. It's the easiest way of making me do something, to tell me that I won't.

I get A's in both RE and biology, just like I said I would. The RE teacher runs up to me and hugs me, thrilled that I've proved her wrong.

The biology teacher doesn't say a word.

The prom, end of year 11. Rach is there. I'm more nervous than I've ever been before a rugby match. *Do it*, I say to myself. *Talk to her. She's right here. It's now or never.*

So I do. We sit on a bench and chat. It's the happiest day of my life, honestly it is.

And that's it. From that moment onwards, I've got no interest in any other girl. I know she's the one for me. She's the one I'm going to marry.

When you know, you know. And I know.

July. I immerse myself in the Lions tour to New Zealand, getting up at stupid o'clock to watch some of the games. Martyn Williams is my hero, and I'm so thrilled when he makes it onto the pitch as a replacement in the third Test, even though both the match and the series are long gone by then. I'm also transfixed by the way Marty Holah at 7 plays for the Maori All Blacks when they beat the Lions before the Test series begins.

The next time my beloved Lions shirt comes back from the wash, I fold it neatly and put it in the bottom of a drawer.

'What's up?' Mum says. 'Don't you like wearing it anymore?'

'Next time I wear that top,' I reply, 'it's going to be the real thing.'

Rach and I start going out. I'm lovesick, quite literally; every time I see her, I'm so nervous that I throw up beforehand. I've only ever been sick before a match once, and even that was just reflex from a cough I had, but with Rachel it happens every time. 'I'm not sure this is normal,' Mum says. Maybe not, I think, but Kyle in *South Park* used to get sick like this too whenever he met a girl, so at least I've got company (even if that company is a cartoon character).

Sometimes it even happens when I'm with Rachel, in the car for example. 'Rach, can you pull over? I just – there's something I need to get behind that post-box.' And then I'm out of the car and chucking my guts up behind the post-box, as if it's two in the morning and I've had a skinful.

If I haven't learned the lesson from last year's case of free golf tuition, I do this time round. I'm playing two years up by now, and we go to face Glantaf. Last time we played them my opposite number started strangling me, and when I fought back he bit my finger. At the next kick-off, I told the fly-half to put it on him, and when he caught it I forearmed him in the face as hard as I could. He never came back at me for the rest of the game.

So there's a bit of history here. I'm thinking about this and looking to see whether this bloke's going to be playing again today, so when I see a Cardiff Blues car parked near the pitch I don't take much notice. I assume they're there to watch one of the Glantaf boys, a big, hard-running back called Jamie Roberts.

Turns out they know all about Jamie, and it's me they've come to watch.

I do well at a Cardiff Blues academy training session and get taken on there. They pay me £50 a month, which for a teenage boy is the dog's bollocks. No paper round, protein shakes whenever I want, travel expenses too. Happy days.

Not quite. The coach is really down on me, giving me three or four out of 10 when I know I've played much better than that. Not just one game or two, but every single time. Maybe he's trying to motivate me, but if so there are better ways of going about it. I'm not a professional player, not yet. I'm a schoolboy who like all teenagers keeps a lot of insecurities tucked away behind the façade. *Am I good enough? Am I tough enough? Am I wasting my time here?*

Just as bad, he keeps putting me in the second row. I'm not a second row. I'm a 7. That's where I play, that's where I'm best.

One night, after another three out of 10 in the second row, I come home in tears. I go straight to the multigym and smash out as hard a session as I can manage, way harder than normal. I'm at it for an hour and a half, fuelled by rage and frustration, pumping weights until I can't move my arms, screaming at the walls.

'Sam!' It's Mum. She's standing by the door. I don't know how long she's been there. 'Sam, what's going on?'

I tell her. She takes me inside the house and calms me down.

The next day, I realise something: the lesson that both this incident and the golf coach have taught me.

Not everyone has my best interests at heart, and not everyone's going to play fair. The only way to deal with it is to make myself so good that they can't do anything other than pick me, and pick me where I play best.

The only person who sets my boundaries is me.

I play for Wales Under-16s that year. Not at 7, ironically, but at 8, which is the next best thing. I don't mind 8 – most of the skills are transferable. It's still the back row, and I'm a back-row player.

On Friday nights, our mates start to go out into Cardiff, and they invite Ben and me along. We usually say no. Because we've always had each other, because we've never needed to bike over to someone's house to find someone to play with, we've never really needed anyone else.

Besides, Fridays are when my granddad Keith comes round, and we sit there watching Friday night sport on TV. Wrestling, boxing, football, rugby league, whatever. Me and Ben and Dad and Keith, while Mum and our elder sister Holly roll their eyes at these cavemen on the sofa.

*   *   *

Dad introduces me to heavy metal. Specifically, he introduces me to Anthrax; and even more specifically, to their track *Refuse to Be Denied*.

Refuse to be denied.

Refuse to compromise.

I listen to it while running the streets at night. Seven – that number again – seven words in the chorus that sum up my entire philosophy.

Refuse to be denied.

Refuse to compromise.

I never stop trying to get better.

On Saturday mornings I watch Super Rugby on TV. I sit there with pen and paper, and whoever's playing 7 – Richie McCaw, George Smith, Schalk Burger – I note down everything they do in the game. Tackles, rucks, carries, turnovers. In the afternoon I play for the Blues Under-16s, and when we're given our own statistics for the match I compare them to those of the pros. So I might get something like eight tackles, 16 rucks, eight carries and no turnovers, while McCaw would be on 21 tackles, 40 rucks, 18 carries and five turnovers.

You've got a bit of a way to go here, old son, I think to myself.

But having a way to go doesn't matter if I'm on the right path. I start jackalling – trying to steal the ball at the point of contact – in school matches, just like I've seen McCaw do. No one else my age is doing that. They don't even know what jackalling is; they just tackle and ruck.

One of my teachers, Steve Williams, was a flanker for Neath, so he does one-on-one breakdown training with me too. It all helps me improve.

Ben and I play for Welsh Schools together. He's a fabulous player, in many ways better than me, and that's not false modesty on my part. He plays at outside centre, and his foot-work and handling are absolutely brilliant. His hero is Brian O'Driscoll, and it shows.

One match, he suffers a shoulder injury, and a freakishly bad one too: serious nerve damage. The doctors tell him that continuing to play is really risky, and that the injury's only going to get worse under contact. Besides, he wants to be a physio, and for that he needs strength in his upper body.

He's 16 years old, and his rugby career is over. I couldn't be more gutted if it had happened to me. Rugby is something we both live for, something we share. I feel his pain, his anguish and his frustration as though they were all mine.

From now on, I resolve, I'm going to play every game not just for me but for Ben too. I will carry his career, the one he didn't have, in my heart and on the crest of my jersey. I will achieve the things he couldn't, not because he wasn't capable but because he wasn't given the opportunity.

2006. After about a year, I manage to stop throwing up when-ever I see Rach. It's such a relief when this happens.

'Sam,' Rach says.

'What?'

'I think it's time you met my parents.'

And the throwing up starts all over again.

* * *

Rach challenges me to a game of badminton. She's playing for the Wales senior team by now, so I know she's pretty good, but I reckon I can have her. I'm taller, quicker, more powerful, and I've got good hand–eye co-ordination. This might even be quite easy, I think.

It is easy. It's 21–0.

To her.

She does me up like a kipper, hook, line and sinker. There's not a single rally that lasts more than three shots. She's always one step ahead of me, teeing me up one side and then putting the shuttlecock the other, or driving me deep to the back of the court before dropping it just over the net. I'm sweating and swearing and throwing my racket. There are a bunch of kids watching, and they're all laughing: look at Sam Warburton, being beaten by a girl.

It's the way you're moving, Rach says. You're turning like a boat, slow and cumbersome. Watch my feet. Look at the shuffle, quick steps side to side. You don't need to keep twisting your body this way and that.

Right, I say. Race over 10 metres. I'll definitely beat you.

Ten metres there, ten metres back, she replies.

No way, I say. She's so much smaller than me that she'll turn much quicker, and any advantage I have in straight-line speed will be cancelled out.

Finally she agrees just to the ten metres there, and I do beat her.

We play tennis on holiday. I beat her. We play again. She beats me.

That's 2–2 in the Warburton–Thomas Cup. We agree to leave it there for the sake of our relationship. Otherwise in a few years' time we'll be going to the lawyers, and when they ask why we're getting divorced we'll both simultaneously say 'sport'.

2007. Ben and I opt for the same A levels: chemistry, biology and PE. We revise together, and make it count; not the usual 'Oh, I spent ten hours in the library' stuff, conveniently forgetting that half that time was coffee and chat, but constructive and regimented, applying the principles of rugby training to revision. Half an hour on, ten minutes off, and repeat. Work out targets for sessions and stick to them.

A couple of months before the exams, I get a phone call. The bloke says he's from the Welsh Rugby Union, and can he ask me a few questions. Sure, I say.

'Where's your dad from?' he asks.

'Originally? London. But his folks are from Lancashire.'

'Like Warburton's bread?'

'Exactly.'

'And your mum?'

'Born in Somerset. Her folks are Welsh, but her great-grand-father had Scottish roots.' My full name is Sam Kennedy-Warburton – the Kennedy is Mum's side, and since she has a sister and their parents were both only children, she wants to keep the name alive – but I don't use it too often when playing as it's a bit of a mouthful and makes me sound way too posh.

'Right,' he says. 'Thanks.'

Now he knows that I'm eligible to play for England and Scotland as well as Wales. Sure, I've played all my representative rugby for Wales at age-group level, but that doesn't matter. You can play senior rugby for any country you're eligible for, and the moment you have your first cap that's it, you can't play for anyone else (at least not without taking three years out to qualify for another country). *Shit, better cap this kid quick*: that's what the bloke from the WRU's thinking.

Sure enough, a week or so later I get asked to play for Wales in the World Sevens Series at Twickenham.

It's a great honour, but I turn it down. First, I don't want it to interfere with my exams, and second, I'm carrying a knock on my knee. But I assure the WRU that they don't need to worry about me turning out with a red rose or a thistle on my chest. I'm Welsh through and through, and I'll never play for anyone else.

LEADERSHIP 1: PERSONALITY

It might sound obvious, but one of the first rules of leadership is this: know who you are. There are as many different styles of leadership as there are personality types, and trying to adopt one that doesn't suit you is not just pointless but counterproductive.

The WRU once asked us all to take personality tests based on the Myers–Briggs model. These tests assess personality in four main areas:

- How you focus attention or get your energy (Extraversion/ Introversion)
- How you perceive or take in information (Sensing/Intuition)
- How you prefer to make decisions (Thinking/Feeling)
- How you orient yourself to the external world (Judgement/ Perception)

You're assigned to one category in each area, which means there are 16 possible personality types. I came out as ISFJ: introverted, sensing, feeling and judging.

Introverted people tend to be quiet, reserved, and generally prefer either being alone or with a few close friends rather than a wide circle of acquaintances. They find that large social situations sap energy from them rather than give energy to them. This is why I was the quiet kid on the bus to Bridgend, why I preferred Friday nights in with Ben, my dad and my granddad, and why I bunked off the end-of-year prom!

Sensing people tend to be more concrete than abstract in their thinking, focusing on facts and details rather than ideas and concepts. Hence my choice of A levels, all science-based one way or another rather than arts or humanities, and why I liked to collect data on players while watching Super 15 matches. I was always the kind of player who would do the groundwork first and never try to wing it.

Feeling people tend to value personal considerations above objective criteria. My parents brought me up with strong values, especially as regards treating other people. For example, I would defend kids against bullies even if it made me look bad in the eyes of my mates.

Judging people like to plan things, make decisions a long way ahead of time, and try to ensure that things are as predictable as possible by leaving little to chance. I always liked to prepare the best I could for any test, be it a rugby match or an exam.

ISFJs are often known as Protectors or Defenders, and I fit the broader characteristics of the personality type too. Here are a dozen ISFJ traits that apply to me.

- I have a strong work ethic, which sometimes means that I take too much on.
- I feel responsible towards others and like to help by sharing my knowledge, experience, time and energy with anyone who needs it.
- I like to be conscientious and methodical, to do jobs to the best of my ability, and to see them through to the end.

- I like working within established structures and organisations.
- I'm deeply devoted to my family and value long-term friendships.
- I can be reserved with people I don't know well, which can sometimes be misread as standoffish.
- I don't like to draw attention to myself, and prefer to work behind the scenes rather than out front.
- I don't seek out positions of authority.
- I work well on my own.
- I'm receptive to new ideas.
- I can take things personally even if they're not meant that way, and find it hard to wall off my professional life from my personal one.
- I don't like confrontation (at least off the pitch!) and will try to avoid it wherever possible, always seeking to build consensus rather than laying down the law.

All of these traits fed into my leadership style, as you'll see throughout this book. For example, I was never one for big, rousing speeches or putting myself in front of the camera; I went out of my way to try and get to know the newer boys in the squad; and I felt more comfortable as time went by and I knew the nucleus of the team better.

But what worked for me wouldn't have worked for other people, because their personalities were different from mine. Leadership only works if your personality informs the way you carry out those leadership duties rather than vice versa. Know yourself, and you'll know how best you can lead.

2

TOYOTA STADIUM, CHICAGO

41.8623°N, 87.6167°W

Saturday, 6 June 2009. Wales v USA

The USA kick off, Ryan Jones catches it, is hit in the tackle – and is knocked out. Literally in the first minute. I'm on the bench as back-row cover. If Ryan comes off, I'm on. Robin turns to me. 'Get ready.'

Ryan doesn't come off immediately. He stays on, hoping that if he's out there long enough he'll recover. Am I coming on or not? Ryan doesn't look too great, but it's not my call.

Thoughts whirl through my head. What do you want? To come on at 50, like you presumed you would? Or now, before you have time to think about it? Are you ready? Doesn't matter. You have to be ready when they need you.

With 19 minutes gone, Robin and the medics have seen enough. Ryan's groggy and not playing anywhere like he usually does.

Off he comes. On I go. There's more than an hour left to play.

This is it. I'm a Wales player now, and no one can take that away from me.

2007. I'm playing for Glamorgan Wanderers when I tear my hamstring. It keeps me out of the whole of Wales's 2008 Under-20s Six Nations campaign. It's pretty much the first time I've ever been injured, certainly badly enough to keep me out for a match or two. It feels like the end of the world, watching my body waste away while I have to rest and let nature take its course. As if all the good work I've put in so far has been for nothing.

Injury #1. It won't be my last, not by any means.

2008. 'You should get an agent.' That's what I hear time and again. A couple of the other academy boys have already got people interested in them, and of course a lot of the senior Blues players have them already. I get a few names recommended to me, and a few calls from agents sounding me out. They're all slick and have the sales patter down to a tee, but I bide my time. I want an agent who's out for me more than for himself, who's going to look to manage my career in the long term rather than just getting as much money as possible up front.

Then I meet Derwyn. He used to be a player himself – 19 Welsh caps and more than 150 games for Cardiff – so he knows the system and what the game demands.

'What do you want to achieve?' he asks. I've heard him ask this of some of the other boys at the academy too, and they all answer the same way. *I want to turn professional. I want to play regional. I want to play for Wales.*

'I want to be the best 7 in the world,' I say.

He doesn't laugh or make a face. Just says he can help me do exactly that.

I sign with him. It's one of the best moves I'll ever make.

* * *

First day training with the senior Blues squad. I grew up with a Blues season ticket: watch them at the Arms Park on Friday night, play for Whitchurch on Saturday morning. All that time, I'd dreamed about making the jump from one to the other. And now I've done it.

You're good enough to be here, I tell myself. *They wouldn't have signed you if they didn't think you were up to it.*

'Hello, Sam.'

It's Martyn Williams: club captain, Wales legend, and my rugby hero. Also current holder of the Blues and Wales number 7 shirt. He was one of the main reasons why I wanted to play rugby. I remember watching the 2005 Six Nations and not a game would go by where he wouldn't get man of the match or score a try. He was absolutely amazing.

He shakes my hand – the very first person to do so at the club – and takes me under his wing.

This is one of the bittersweet things about rugby, that you can end up competing for the same position as someone you idolised as a schoolboy, and maybe even usurping them. Right now, that's a way off, but it won't be for long.

And maybe Martyn sees it before I do. Later, he'll tell me: 'I knew you were going to take my spot as soon as you walked in. I saw you training and I knew, Christ, I haven't got long left here.'

September. I'm feeling good. I might have missed the Under-20s Six Nations, but I was back in the side – captaining the side, in fact – for the summer Junior World Cup, where we reached the semi-final. I've just signed for the Blues, my first pro contract. It's the last pre-season game, and I'm playing well.

Then I go over on my shoulder. It's weird, because there's no pain, but when I press the bone it bounces.

You've detached your collarbone, the physios say. The ligaments have gone round the ACJ, the acromioclavicular joint. It doesn't hurt because there's no nerve damage there. But you have to let it heal.

You've also got a hairline fracture of the knee, which will need an operation, so this is as good a time to do it as any.

How long?

Five months.

Five months?!

Injury #2.

The Blues boys are very sympathetic. They put Natasha Bedingfield's *I Bruise Easily* – or *Warby's Song*, as it's now known – on the gym stereo at full volume.

According to the Swiss-American psychiatrist Elisabeth Kübler-Ross, there are five stages of grief: denial, anger, bargaining, depression and acceptance. Clearly no injury, no matter how bad, is on the same scale as a genuine bereavement, but the same five stages apply in both cases.

Denial kicks in more or less the moment I get injured. *It isn't that bad. The pain will wear off soon. I didn't even fall that badly. How can I be injured when I'm in such good condition?*

Once the medical staff have made their diagnosis, that's when anger kicks in. *This is so unfair. Someone else will come into the team, take my place and play so well that I'll never get it back. I've got all this energy and I have to sit here like a little old man. It's all I want to do, play rugby. Is that too much to ask? Oh – and it hurts. It really hurts.*

I can't stay angry forever, though. The anger subsides and gives way to rationalisation, which brings with it bargaining. *If I do all my rehab, then I'll get back to where I was. If only I can get back in time for this match, then I don't mind missing a few less important ones further down the line. I'll swap this cruciate ligament injury for a couple of ankle strains.*

And when the bargaining doesn't work, which of course it doesn't, that's when the depression comes. *I'm stuck on my own in the gym while the rest of the boys are training and playing. I'm on the outside of the squad looking in, part of it but not part of it. Sportsmen don't like injury, because injury means weakness, and when they see it they move away in case it infects them too. Every day is such a slog. I'm not making progress quickly enough.*

But I won't be a pro player for very long if I let the depression and moping linger. This is where the acceptance comes in. *Everyone gets injured. There are always silver linings to things. I can work on different aspects of my fitness. I can take a mental break from the relentless grind.*

These stages don't always happen in strict sequence, they don't all last the same amount of time, and they won't remain constant throughout my career. Right now, when I'm still young and inexperienced, the anger and frustration last longer and feel more acute. Later on, when I'm more used to being injured and more secure in my place in the team, I'll be able to get to acceptance much more quickly.

Friday, 3 April 2009. My first game for the Blues is a Magners League fixture up in Edinburgh. Early April, a bit of a nothing match on most fronts. We're mid-table only six weeks from the end of the season, and we've rested two-thirds of our first team ahead of the Heineken Cup quarter-final next week. The match is nothing to write home about: one of those stop-start affairs with no real fluency. Edinburgh win 16–3.

A bit of a nothing match for everybody but me, that is. I'm excited to play, of course, but I'm still only 20 and it shows. It's not that I play badly; more that I'm not strong enough. I've never played against people of this calibre before, and I feel a bit out of my depth. I'm used to being among the most physically imposing players on any team, and it's a shock to find myself being muscled off the ball time and again. My opponents are gnarly and grizzled; they know all the tricks, all the body positions, all the little niggles out of the ref's sight. I'm a greenhorn.

There's only one solution, the same one there's always been. Work. Work harder. Work smarter.

I've only played a handful of games for the Blues when I get the call-up. *The* call-up, that is: the Wales summer tour to Canada and the USA.

It feels both weird and entirely normal. Weird, in that I'm still only 20 and pretty inexperienced at senior level; but normal, in that if I'm going to be the best 7 in the world then I have to start playing for my country sooner or later.

It's the first time I've ever flown business class. I'm like a kid in a sweet shop: the seats, the films, the food. All the way over, I keep sneaking a peek at the official tour guide, and my head shot in it. I try to act cool. Not sure how well I succeed.

Four years ago, men like Dwayne Peel and Ryan Jones were playing for the Lions against the All Blacks, and I was watching them on TV on Saturday mornings. Now they're sitting alongside me. For them, this tour's a step down from what they're used to. For me, it's just the opposite. I remind myself that they were in my position once: the newbie, the hopeful.

I keep my head down, as far as possible. I don't know many people, I'm conscious that I've got a lot to learn, and I'm also feeling homesick. It's only a two-week tour, but when you've spent all your life living either at home or within half a mile of it, that's a long time to be several thousand miles away.

I sit in the team room and watch what the others are doing, looking to pick up pointers as to how senior pros handle themselves and prepare for matches. *Be like a sponge. Soak it all up.*

Saturday, 30 May. Our first match is against Canada. I'm a sub, which is always much harder than starting. When you're starting, you know your timings and you can work backwards off them. When you're a sub, all that's out of the window. You might be on in the first minute, or the fiftieth, or not at all. If you use an energy gel, when do you take it? Too early or too late, and it won't be effective. The starting XV have first dibs on strapping and so on in the dressing-room, which is of course entirely right, but it does mean that the subs can feel rushed in their own preparations. Everything's a little bit out of sync when you're a sub, basically.

We make reasonably heavy weather of the game. At one stage, not long after half-time, it's 16–16, and we have to work hard to get more than one score ahead and close it out 32–23. All through the second half I'm waiting for coach Robin McBryde to give me the nod. There are seven of us on the bench, and one by one they go on until it's just me and Nicky Robinson left. Canada have emptied their bench, but we're still sitting there like lemons.

Two minutes left, and the game looks safe. *Come on*, I think. *Give me a runout. Even if I don't touch the ball or make a tackle, at least I'll have got it over with. Good or bad, long or short, it doesn't matter.*

For almost 80 minutes I've been on edge, warming up now and then, trying not to get ahead of myself but still being ready for anything.

It never happens. The final whistle goes, and I'm still on the bench. What a comedown. After all that, what a massive anti-climax. I feel like crying. I've got so much energy that I could run round the pitch non-stop for all of those 80 minutes I didn't get to play.

That night, on the phone to Mum, I do cry. I let all my frustration flow out while she listens and does her best to comfort me.

'Mum,' I say, 'can you put Ted on?'

Ted's my dog. He's a rough collie, and he's named after Teddy Sheringham, one of my Spurs heroes. He's very vocal, and he likes to talk to me: howling and woofing and barking when I make noises. His favourite sounds are the theme tune to *Coronation Street* and the sound of an ice-cream van, so I sit in my room in Toronto and sing these down the phone to him. Ted howls them back to me, which makes me start crying all over again.

Saturday, 6 June. One week later. We're playing the USA at Toyota Stadium in Chicago. Again I'm on the bench, and I'm thinking that if I don't get on this time I'm going to explode. Surely they'll bring me on? What would be the point of taking me all the way to North America and not giving me any game time?

Eight and a half thousand miles away, though I'm only very dimly aware of it, the British and Irish Lions are playing Free State on their tour of South Africa.

Here in Chicago, the USA kick off, Ryan catches it, is hit in the tackle – and is knocked out. Literally in the first minute. I'm back-row cover. If Ryan comes off, I'm on. Robin turns to me. 'Get ready.'

Ryan doesn't come off immediately. He stays on, hoping that if he's out there long enough he'll recover. Am I coming on or not? Ryan doesn't look too great, but it's not my call.

Thoughts whirl through my head. *What do you want? To come on at 50, like you presumed you would? Or now, before you have time to think about it? Are you ready? Doesn't matter. You have to be ready when they need you.*

With 19 minutes gone, Robin and the medics have seen enough. Ryan's groggy and not playing anywhere like he usually does. Off he comes. On I go. There's more than an hour left to play. This is it. I'm a Wales player now, and no one can take that away from me.

Blimey, it's quick. Doesn't matter that this is 'only' the USA, who are a rung or two down from the highest echelons of world rugby, and doesn't matter that we run out easy winners, 48–15. It's noticeably quicker than the Heineken Cup, which is itself noticeably quicker than the Magners League. It's as though someone's running it at normal speed plus a half. The passes, the runners, the tackles, all coming fast and relentless, and I have to concentrate more fiercely than ever before just to keep up.

That concentration and the physical effort take their toll – even though I didn't play the first 20 minutes, I find myself cramping up with 10 minutes to go, which I find out later happens to lots of new caps as they get used to the pace of the game – but I play pretty well.

Back at the hotel, I find myself in the lift with team manager Alan Phillips.

'You had a good game out there,' he says.

'Thank you.'

'You know what I think? I think we've found the next Martyn Williams.'

Friday, 16 October. There's a bug going round the Blues camp before we play a Heineken Cup match away to Sale Sharks. I've got it too, a bad chest infection, but even though I'm an international player now I still feel too young to assert myself properly. So I play. I feel terrible, and I play even worse than that. I give away two tries all on my own.

It's the worst professional game I'll ever play, but it teaches me another lesson: illness is as bad as an injury, so treat it like one. If you've got the flu or the shits, pull yourself out. The fans won't know that you're crook, and they won't care either. You're not doing yourself, your team or your reputation any favours. This isn't playing for the local second XV, making up the numbers or filling in for a mate. This is your livelihood now. If you're not there, you can't play badly.

Friday, 13 November. My second cap against Samoa, but in many ways it feels like my first proper match: my first start, my first playing at 7, my first at home. Samoa have history in Cardiff – they won World Cup matches here in both 1991 (when they were called 'Western Samoa', leading to lots of resigned jokes about how it was lucky we hadn't played the whole of Samoa) and 1999.

Just over one minute gone. We break through the middle and Dwayne feeds me on the inside. There's no defender in front of me and for a split second I sense glory, but in the next stride David Lemi tackles me and then knocks the ball from my grasp just as I'm about to pop it up to Huw Bennett. Another reminder of how narrow the margins are at this level. In a club match, I could well have been in under the posts.

It's a scrappy game – we're playing in our change yellow kit, which doesn't feel at all Welsh – and though we win 17–13, we should close it out much earlier than we do. I play pretty well, though a knock-on reminds me that Ben was right when he said my handling needs to improve, and like most of our forwards I seem to spend half the match clinging onto Henry Tuilagi, who's basically a wrecking ball in a blue shirt and the hardest guy to tackle I've ever come across.

The next day, I'm going up an escalator in the St David's 2 shopping centre when I hear someone saying, 'That's Sam Warburton.' Rach and I try not to laugh, not because it's not flattering but because it feels a bit weird. No one's ever said 'That's Sam Warburton' before. It's the first tiny taste of something I'll have to get used to over the years: not of being famous, because I genuinely don't think that's a word that can ever be applied to me, but of being locally well recognised.

Saturday, 28 November. I come off the bench against Australia. The match is memorable for two reasons.

First, Australia hammer us, scoring three tries in the first 25 minutes, and – though obviously I don't yet know it – it's the start of a miserable personal run in a Welsh shirt against Australia. By the time my career comes to an end I'll have played for Wales against Australia ten times, and lost the lot.

Second, when I come on it's in place of my mate Dan Lydiate – Lyds – which means I end up playing blindside with Martyn Williams at openside. Or rather, we play as twin opensides. Rather than having a six who's a carrier and a seven who's a scavenger, we both do a bit of each, and spell each other if need be. After a particularly draining period of play, Martyn asks me if I'll jump on the openside for the next scrum just so he can catch his breath, and I'm happy to do so.

'This is the way forward,' Gethin Jenkins says afterwards. 'Playing two opensides. Makes you as a team so quick to the breakdown.'

He's right, of course. When it comes to rugby, Gethin usually is. He reads the game so well, and he isn't afraid to speak his mind either; he's the only player I've ever seen grab the water-boy's mike and yell up to the coaches, 'Get X off now, he's playing shit!' (X *was* playing shit, and the coaches did indeed pull him off.)

In years to come this is how I'll play with Justin Tipuric for Wales and Sean O'Brien for the Lions; I might have 6 on my back, but I'll still be playing as a 7. And those combinations will respectively yield two of the most memorable victories of my international career.

Sunday, 17 January 2010. The Six Nations is almost upon us, and I know this is it. Summer tours and autumn internationals can be experimental – a chance to try out new players and combinations, perhaps give the more senior and experienced players a rest – but the Six Nations is the real thing. Every country picks their best team. If I'm selected here, I'll really start to feel that I belong in a Welsh shirt.

Even as a fan, I always loved the Six Nations, and on the morning of every match I'd read all the papers I could find: the predictions, the stories, the latest bulletins from inside the Wales camp. The tournament has such a long and varied history, and every year the players get a chance to add to that history by making some of their own. Five weekends to look forward to in the cold and damp winter days, and the simple primary colours of the competing teams: Welsh red, English white, Irish green, French blue, Scottish navy and Italian azure.

I'm driving back from Loughborough, where I've been seeing Rach. She's studying there, and it's 150 miles each way, but we try to see each other as much as possible. I know the squad's due to be announced today, and each player selected will receive a text message by midday to let them know.

I've got my ringer turned up to max as midday approaches. Silence.

The midday news on the radio comes and goes. Still nothing.

Maybe I didn't play well enough in the autumn internationals. Maybe I haven't been playing sufficiently well for the Blues lately. I think I've done enough on both those fronts, but then again I'm not the one making the selection calls. Am I another nearly man? Rugby's full of them. The kind who play a few games at international level but can't really cut it.

At 12.15 I pull into a petrol station. I'm filling the car up when I hear the text tone.

Congratulations, you're in the Six Nations squad. An email will follow.

The relief. The sheer relief. 'Yeah!' I shout as loud as I can. The other customers are looking at me a bit strangely.

The attendant's voice comes over the tannoy. 'Pump 6. No mobile phones on the forecourt.'

Saturday, 13 February. Wales 14 Scotland 24, with 12 minutes left. I come on for Martyn. All the second half we've been attacking, and even though we're still ten points down, we – and the crowd – believe we can come back. The game's frantic, and I have to hit the ground running, adjust myself to its pace instantly.

I make some yards down the left-hand side. A minute or so later, I'm caught in possession by a couple of Scottish forwards. I'm fresh against some tired boys, and I'm hitting the rucks well, but I'm not carrying the ball as well as I could do.

There are only three minutes left when Pence – Leigh Halfpenny – scoots in for a try, which Stephen Jones converts. As we go back to halfway, Jonathan Thomas says something, but although he's right next to me I can't hear a word over the crowd.

We still trail by three. Now Lee Byrne goes through, kicks ahead – and is taken out by Phil Godman, who's sin-binned. Penalty. Three points to draw. Stephen knocks it over as though it's the training ground.

This is fantastic. If this is the Six Nations, I can't get enough of it.

The clock's already gone red when Scotland kick off for the last time. With Godman and Scott Lawson in the bin, we've got a two-man advantage. Stephen kicks to the corner for Pence to chase. Pence scrabbles, darts, sets up the ruck. We work it left and left again – and there's Shane Williams, arm aloft as he goes under the posts to win it in the second minute of added time.

The Millennium goes mental.

There's this guy called Andy McCann, who's working with the squad. He's a psychologist, which of course immediately brings to mind patients on couches and drawings of a house that reveals you have unresolved mother-attachment issues or something like that.

Andy gets that kind of stereotyping a lot, and always explains patiently that psychoanalysts, not psychologists, are the couch and Freud guys. He likes to think of himself more as a mental-skills coach, in the same way that we have coaches for attack, defence, scrums, fitness and so on. And it's about something physical that I first really get chatting to him.

'I've got some confidence issues when it comes to ball-carrying,' I say.

'That's what I'm here for,' he replies.

I go to see him in his room. He doesn't tell me which other members of the team he works with, as all his stuff is confidential: more like a doctor–patient relationship than a coach–player one. I know that about half the squad use him, but I don't know which half unless boys come out and say so. There's still a stigma attached to seeing him in some quarters, as though it's embarrassing, an admission of weakness.

I don't care. Everyone can improve somewhere, and I'm no different. I want to be a better player tomorrow than I was yesterday, and if Andy can help me in that, then happy days. To me, it's no different from doing extra gym training or sitting in my pyjamas counting McCaw's tackle rate in Super Rugby. If it's going to give me an advantage, then I'd be a fool not to give it a go.

In any case, Andy instantly makes me feel so comfortable that there's no chance of being embarrassed.

'Breathe in and out,' he says. 'In and out properly, using your diaphragm, until you feel relaxed. When you're breathing in, that's positive green energy; when you're breathing out, that's negative red energy. Positive energy in, negative energy out. Good. Close your eyes. Now, your next game's against Ireland at Croke Park, yes? Imagine the noise. So much noise. Always is with Irish crowds, the way they get behind their team. You're on the bench, and all this noise is swirling around you. Embrace it. Don't let it intimidate you. It's there for you just as much as it is the Irish players. Use it, the way they use it. Feed off it, the way they feed off it.

'You're warming up. Along the sidelines, behind the posts. Getting your head as well as your body right. Any minute now you're going to get the nod. There it is. Warby, you're on. The announcer's voice. 'Wales, Number 19, Sam Warburton. The crowd cheering your name. On you come. You're relaying instructions from the coaches. Your voice and body language scream energy and freshness, and those by themselves give the other lads a lift.

'First play after you've come on. You've got the ball. Short pass off 9. Now, don't think of it from your point of view. Think of it from the point of view of the Irish player waiting to tackle you. What's he seeing? He's seeing how big you are, how strong, how dynamic. He's seeing all your explosive power, and how much you love the confrontation, and he knows that when you smash into him it's going to hurt and it's going to take him backwards, and bang! There it is, and you're through him and there are a couple of your boys piling in behind and you've got front-foot ball and the Irish are scrambling and your backs love you for setting them up like this.

'OK. Rewind back to the moment you get the ball. Now imagine it from the ref's point of view. Imagine where he's standing, looking at you from side-on. He's seeing the determination on your face, and all that power in you as you run, and he's thinking "I'd better have my eyes peeled here, because this boy's going to be hard to put down" – and bang! You're through the first tackle – which means he'll be giving Wales good ball, which means Ireland will try to slow it down at the ruck, which means they're going to risk getting pinged for infringing at the breakdown.

'OK. Rewind again to the pass off 9. Now imagine yourself in the crowd, high in the stands. What have you come to watch? The hits. Think of the ancient Romans and the gladiators. It's alpha males, it's one-on-one dominance. It's in our DNA. The crowd see your power and intent, and they're bracing themselves for something they can feel 25 rows back – and bang! They shudder at the impact, and then they're looking at each other and grinning, like "How about that!"'

We do this for four separate incidents – a carry, a lineout, a tackle and a jackal. For each incident Andy makes me think of it from the same three viewpoints: the opposition player, the ref and the crowd. By the time we've done all 12, I'm feeling so confident that I could run out at Croke Park here and now. I see it all unfolding almost in slow motion, as though my brain and body are so much quicker than everybody else's.

I open my eyes.

'How long do you reckon we've been in here?' he asks.

'Ten minutes?'

'Thirty-five.'

Andy helps me in other ways too. He teaches me relaxation techniques, tensing and relaxing various parts of my body until they feel heavy. He'll massage my head and neck until I'm practically asleep. And he works with me to produce a document that we call *Warby's Winning Ways*.

It's ten pages or so, and I keep it as a PDF on my phone. It's there so that I can continue to reinforce my positive mindset and remind myself that I'm good enough to be playing international rugby, that I deserve to be playing international rugby and that I add value to every team I play for.

On the front is a picture of me walking out of the tunnel at the Millennium before a Wales match. Behind me the tunnel is lit up all red, and on my face is an expression of total focus: confident in my ability, completely ready for the battle ahead.

Inside are some of my statistics on the pitch and in the gym: I'm strong, I'm fit, no one's going to better me physically. There are positive newspaper clippings from people in the game I respect praising me. There are photographs of me playing well, and of people who matter to me: my parents, my brother and sister, Rach, Mr Morris and Lennox Lewis, whom I idolised as a kid. My dogs Ted and Gus too, of course; wouldn't be properly Warby without my dogs.

We've even included pictures and logos of the companies that sponsor me, such as Land Rover, adidas and PAS supplements, because these companies wouldn't be endorsing me if they didn't believe in me both on and off the pitch.

Later in my career, when I'm more confident as a player, a person and a captain, I won't need all this. But right now the third of those isn't yet an issue, and the first two still need a lot of work. So I keep *Warby's Winning Ways* close by at all times, and it's invaluable.

Saturday, 20 March. My first Six Nations start, against Italy at the Millennium. My opposite number is Mauro Bergamasco. He's smaller than me, but he's a very good player with that bit of devil in him that all top opensides need. *Un cane sciolto*, as he once described himself: a marauding dog, an outlaw. He's played on the wing and at scrum-half for them too. Definitely not your average 7.

'If you don't get the first shot in on him,' Martyn tells me before the match, 'he'll niggle you all game.'

I don't need telling twice.

Five minutes in, I see Mauro contesting a ruck. I come flying in like an Exocet and clear him right out. He, the ref, the crowd – they all see and feel that, just like Andy told me they would.

Mauro doesn't come back at me all game.

* * *

Of all the things I work on and am known for, the breakdown is the single most important aspect. It's a much bigger part of the game than it used to be; there are something like 170 breakdowns every game, which is almost double the number at the 1995 World Cup, which marked the end of the amateur era, and almost six times the number back in the early 1970s. There are also four and a half times as many breakdowns per game nowadays than scrums and lineouts combined.

That's helped a new species of defender evolve: the jackal, who pounces on the ball when it's taken into contact by the opposition and tries to scavenge it. The ultimate aim is of course the turnover, when you rip the ball from the opposition player and secure it for your own side. An interception try apart, the turnover is the single biggest momentum shifter in rugby. Suddenly, the team that were attacking not only have the wind knocked out of them by the frustration of losing the ball, but they also have to instantly reorganise into a defensive structure before the counterattack comes – and, statistically, that moment of transition leads to a disproportionate number of scoring opportunities. A player who can reliably secure four or five turnovers a game is worth his weight in gold.

In every team I play for, I am that player.

The jackal is the one who comes in after the tackler to try and grab the ball from the man on the floor. If you're exceptionally quick you can be both tackler and jackal, bouncing up off the floor to go from one to the other, as long as you release the opponent after the tackle and before the attempted jackal. But at international level things happen so fast that this isn't usually an option. Better to hunt in pairs, as I do with Lyds; he goes low to bring the man down and I'm on that man in a flash. Lyds and me: tackle and jackal.

The jackal's not allowed to support his own bodyweight, which means no knee resting on the opposition player or hands on the ground beyond the ball. This means I have to be both very flexible and very strong; very flexible to get into the low, wide stance I need to secure the ball, and very strong to withstand the hits coming in from the other opposition players arriving at the ruck. Sometimes you get smacked by two or three men at a single ruck. It hurts. Trust me.

So for 15 minutes before and after every training session, I work exclusively on hip mobility: working my glutes, my groin and my hamstrings. I take the heaviest kettlebell I can find, set myself in a sumo squat and go from left to right and back again, shifting my weight all the way over onto one foot and then back through the centre to the other. Deep and strong, I tell myself. Deep and strong.

It's basic physics. The lower you can go, the harder you are to shift. As Vince Lombardi, the legendary American football coach, used to tell his blockers, 'The low man wins.' If you're low enough over the ball, the opposition players won't be able to get beneath you to drive you up and out of the way. That's where the leverage comes in, and without that they're trying to shift you backwards without first weakening your strong position.

There is one way of getting me out of the jackal position, though only one team have worked it out and even then I'm not sure they know they've done it. Whenever you play against France, you can guarantee they'll be grabbing your balls like it's going out of fashion. That gets me off the ball better than any clean-out. Just pull my bollocks and I'm off.

Sunday, 23 May. The Blues reach the final of the Amlin Challenge Cup, basically the plate competition for those teams that don't make it through to the latter stages of the Heineken Cup. The final's in Marseilles, and we're up against Toulon, a side for whom this is almost a home game – less than an hour's drive away – and who are chock full of international superstars: Jonny Wilkinson, Juan Martín Fernández Lobbe, Tana Umaga and Sonny Bill Williams. The stadium's a sea of black and red, Toulon's colours, with only a few hundred Blues fans in there. We're massive, massive underdogs.

And we win. Against all the odds, we hold out for a 28–21 final score. It's the first time any Welsh club has won a European title. I should be bursting with pride, and for the boys I am, but I don't really feel part of the victory.

It's not just that I only came on as a sub in the final, and didn't play in either the quarters against Newcastle or the semis against Wasps. It's that, much as I love the Blues – and I really do, I'm a one-club man, both as player and fan – I don't play quite as intensely for them as I do for Wales.

I still play to a high standard, don't get me wrong. But when I play for Wales, I'm ruined for days afterwards. The way I play is so physical that if I played for the Blues week in, week out the way I play for Wales a handful of times a year, I'd never be off the physio's table, and I'd be retired by the age of 25. My body just wouldn't take it.

It's an emotional thing as much as a physical one. Getting yourself up for the confrontation on the weekend isn't just a matter of putting on the strapping and going out there. It's a lot of mental strain, a lot of the old Shakespearian stiffening up the sinews. That takes its toll too.

And I'm the kind of player who needs pressure to really perform. With the best will in the world, even a European club final isn't remotely on the same level as a Six Nations match, a World Cup knockout tie or a Lions Test. I need those environments in which to perform my best.

And if this leaves the Blues feeling a little short-changed, then I understand that and to an extent agree with it. But like all players, I'm not a robot.

Saturday, 5 June. South Africa at the Millennium. Martyn's been given the summer off. He's 34, and even his storied career is going to end sooner rather than later. This is your chance, coach Warren Gatland – Gats – tells me. This is your chance to prove to me that you're our best 7. He leaves the second half unspoken: not just for this year but next year too, when the World Cup's taking place in New Zealand. Put down a marker for that tournament.

It's my first time playing South Africa, and I love it. Perhaps more than any other team, they pride themselves on physical confrontation, which suits me just fine. In the first 15 seconds I tackle Joe van Niekerk, their number 8, but I get my head position slightly wrong and cop the most almighty crack in the gob.

I can taste the blood welling up inside my mouth. I take my gumshield out and feel for my teeth, checking that they're all there, but the blow's been so hard that I can't feel them properly.

'Mate,' I say to fellow forward Jonathan Thomas, 'can you check my teeth?'

He has a look. 'Yeah, they're all there. You've got a big old gash, though.'

Gashes are ten a penny. Crack on. I throw myself into contact after contact. It's fast and furious, and when I'm subbed off with a couple of minutes to go we're trailing by only three points, 34–31 down.

'Let's have a look at you,' the doctor says afterwards.

He presses his finger on the underside of my jaw, and I almost go through the ceiling.

'Yup,' he says. 'You've broken your jaw.'

Injury #3.

I need an operation, and they put a metal plate in my jaw. I'm ruled out of the summer tour to New Zealand, which is gutting; I so, so wanted to go down there and prove myself against McCaw, pretty much universally regarded as king of the opensides. And if anyone would appreciate playing 78 minutes with a broken jaw, it's him.

Saturday, 27 November. I get to play against McCaw six months later, though not without another injury scare. Three weeks earlier, I tear my calf while playing against Australia. Injury #4. It's somewhere between a grade 1 and a grade 2, which means I should be out for four or five weeks, which in turn means I'll miss the New Zealand match. If you're an international player, they're the team you want to play: the most famous and successful in the history of the game.

'You can get back in time,' Andy says.

'How?'

'By believing.'

'Really?'

'Really. The right mindset can help you so much.'

I ask Prav Mathema, the Wales team physio, if he's on board with this. I half-expect him to roll his eyes and say it's a load of bunk, but no, he agrees with Andy, 100 per cent.

'All right,' I say. 'Let's do this.'

I pepper Prav with questions about the anatomy of the calf. When I have a picture in my mind of what's beneath my skin, I start to visualise the torn fibres knitting themselves back together again. In my head, I send the positive green breathing energy from my lungs to my arteries, directing blood flow to the affected area and dragging all the damaged red energy back out again where it can't do any more harm.

Four weeks, they said. I'm recovered in two. The fourth injury of my career, but the first time I really see how much difference a positive mindset can make.

We lose the game 37–25, but I feel I match McCaw in our personal duel, just as I'd matched David Pocock in the match against Australia. These two are as good as it gets, so to hold my own against them when I've only just turned 22 is a great confidence boost. Prove to me you're our best 7, Gats had said. I've done that, surely, and a bit more too.

Saturday, 19 March 2011. Our final Six Nations game, against France in the Stade de France. Fifteen minutes in, I have to go off with a knock to the knee.

Injury #5.

I watch from the bench as we lose 28–9.

For the team, it's been a mixed tournament. We lost our first match to England – our eighth defeat on the trot including the summer and autumn internationals – before winning the next three games: Scotland 24–6, Italy 24–16 (including my first try for Wales, running the inside line off James Hook: a 15-metre break that gets longer and involves beating more players with every retelling, as all forwards' tries should do), and Ireland 19–13. We end up fourth with six points, the same as Ireland, but behind them on points difference and tries scored.

More than the results, though, there's a sense that things are changing. Some of the old guard have been phased out, leaving a young team that might not have so much experience, but that has got both talent and the willingness to work together. We've done tons of fitness, strength and conditioning work – perhaps to the detriment of the rugby itself at times – because Gats has his eyes not just on this tournament but on the World Cup too. He thinks we can go far, but to do so we'll need to match our opponents physically as much as anything else.

For me personally, the 2011 Six Nations feels like a triumph. Until the injury against France, I've played every minute of every game, and been consistently good. Almost every newspaper's team of the tournament has me in at 7. To be brutally honest, I feel I should win the official player of the tournament award. This year, however, they've changed the way it's decided, with a shortlist purely from the man of the match winners from the opening four rounds, before the public can vote for the winner. As a result, a couple of Italian players come first and second, even though their team received the wooden spoon.

Don't worry about it, Andy says. These things are subjective, which means they're out of your control. Rugby's not figure skating or gymnastics, where the judges' role is paramount. It doesn't matter whether you win player awards or not. What matters is that you play well enough to be in with a shout, and I've certainly done that.

Monday, 9 May. The season is over, and I'm at home thinking about an upcoming week's holiday in Portugal with Rach.

My mobile rings. I look at the screen.

Gats.

I wonder what he wants. It's not like we speak every day, and there's no Wales match until we play the Barbarians next month. He's not the kind of guy who rings just for a chat. I honestly can't think why he could be ringing.

When I answer, he comes straight to the point.

'I'm calling to see if you'd like to be captain against the Barbarians.'

LEADERSHIP 2: PROFESSIONALISM

When people say that rugby went professional in 1995, what they mean is that from then on players could be paid openly rather than clandestinely, which had been the case under amateurism (or 'shamateurism', as it had long been known). This allowed players to devote themselves full-time to rugby rather than needing to hold down day jobs in other sectors.

But for me, and as Gwyn Morris pointed out back at Whitchurch, 'professionalism' doesn't mean simply being paid to play rugby. In fact, professionalism has little or nothing to do with salary. Professionalism is about giving your very best, using your talent to the maximum and being highly competitive. Professionalism is about how you conduct yourself on and off the pitch: how you behave, how you train, how you prepare yourself. Professionalism is about making yourself not just the kind of player others respect, but the kind of person too. There were plenty of rugby players in the amateur era who behaved professionally, just as there are still some players nowadays who don't, not properly at any rate.

As with other aspects of leadership, professionalism begins with the right mindset. You have to set yourself standards, but not limits; you have to hold yourself to minimum requirements rather than maximum ones. For example, Ben hasn't framed and mounted his Wales Under-16 shirt, as for him it's not a measure of success but of failure: it's not how far he got, but how much further he still had to go. If I hadn't got a Lions shirt, I wouldn't have put up a Wales one.

Gats used to say that 'we should be the best at everything that doesn't require talent. Effort doesn't require talent. Hard work doesn't require talent. We should be the best at hard work.' It's never too early to start this. When I'd train at lunchtimes in Whitchurch, that was professional behaviour, what I needed to do to get better. Round about that time, Mr Morris gave me a referee's rulebook. How many 16-year-old kids had even read one of those, let alone owned one? I turned straight to the sections that were most relevant to me, the ones that covered contact rules. I read these until I knew them off by heart, because they helped me work out how to compete, how to know where the offside line was, and so on. Why bother playing a sport unless you knew the rules inside out? But most people didn't. I did, because it gave me an advantage; and if something gives you an advantage, then you'd be nuts not to take it.

Training was an obvious arena in which I could be professional. I was Mr Preseason: you'd have had to tie me down to stop me training. As Muhammad Ali said: 'The fight is won or lost far away from witnesses – behind the lines, in the gym, and out there on the road – long before I dance under those lights.'

Michael Johnson described it well in his book *Gold Rush*. 'The desire to succeed is extremely important, but it's easy to want to be the best in the world. Drive is more important. It's easy to commit to being the Olympic gold medallist, but not as easy to commit to training 50 per cent harder than you did the year before and to making sacrifices to achieve that goal. It is that drive that causes an individual to work for what he desires. Once I started training, my position was simply that every day was an opportunity for me to get better. So with that in mind, any day I missed training or any day I didn't give 100 per cent of the effort I was capable of giving would have been a missed opportunity.'

And 100 per cent means just that. Professionalism means paying attention to the small things as well as the big ones. Sometimes the analysts would play us the voice of the referee for our next match as we did scrum-machine work, not just to add some match atmosphere to the session but so we could get used to his intonation and rhythm, how long he paused for when issuing instructions to set the scrum, and so on.

I hear academy kids asking how to get a Range Rover, how to get an adidas endorsement, that kind of thing. That's topsy-turvy thinking, and a sign of a mindset and values that are all wrong: putting output above input. The true professional would never ask such questions, as the true professional knows that input comes first both in time and importance. Prepare properly, train properly, play properly, and the remainder will look after itself. I picked my endorsements carefully. I didn't just sign with any company that turned up with a cheque and a photoshoot. I only signed with companies whose products I believed in and which I used anyway, or would have used, without being paid.

Rest is a big part of being a professional. You have to learn to say no. I get so many requests to do stuff, and people have no idea how much it all mounts up. I've got people I haven't seen in years who'll drop me a message out of the blue saying: 'I was just wondering …' Luckily Ben and I have largely the same group of friends, so I can say to him: 'I got a message from X – are you in touch with them anyway?' If he says yes, then maybe I'll do it, but if he's not, and they're just chancing their arm, then I definitely won't.

It's hard, sometimes, because people think they own you. I was doing a Q&A up in Cwmbran once, and a bloke stood up and said: 'What are you doing next Monday?' I said I didn't know off the top of my head. 'Well,' he continued, 'we've got a presentation at our club that day, and I bet you don't turn up, because you professional rugby players are all too big for your boots and have forgotten the grassroots game where you come from.'

His tone really took me aback. I explained that I had a certain amount of community work built into my contract, and on top of that I'd go to local clubs, kids' camps and so on. But I also needed nights at home to rest and do nothing, because that was the professional, disciplined thing to do.

At the end, I was signing autographs and stuff – I never left any of those events until I'd signed for anyone who asked – when this same bloke came up. 'Which rugby club are you from?' I asked him. When he told me, I said: 'Just so you know, I'm never going to come up there, purely because of the way you spoke to me.'

A significant aspect of professionalism is honesty: not making excuses, and owning your mistakes. If everyone in a team does that, the environment is healthy and the team has the best chance of improving. Everyone makes mistakes. The only way not to make a mistake is not to try something in the first place. Making a mistake isn't wrong or unprofessional. What *is* wrong and unprofessional is trying to sweep that mistake under the carpet, because by pretending it never happened you deny yourself the opportunity to learn from it next time round.

When other people see you being honest, it inspires them to follow suit. In one training camp, we had a whole load of protein bars brought in, boxes and boxes of them, which were kept in the gym for the boys to take them when they needed.

At one team meeting, the nutritionist said that we had a problem. He'd catered for each person having two bars per day for the duration of the camp, but now there weren't enough anymore, so someone must have been taking more than their fair share. And he knew who the guilty parties were, as there was a CCTV in the gym and it had all been caught on camera. So if whoever had done it didn't own up right now, they'd be exposed as liars and not team players. A few of the younger guys in the squad immediately fessed up, to gales of laughter from the senior boys.

Yes, the young guys had been taking more than their share, but of course there was no CCTV and we could have got more bars delivered at the drop of a hat. The point was to encourage blokes to be honest with each other and with the team as a whole, and it worked. Own up to something before you get called out on it.

Being professional extends to life outside rugby too; indeed, when you're in the public eye it extends pretty much to everything you say or do, 24/7. You represent the club you play for, you represent your country, and you represent the hopes of all the supporters who'd give anything to do what you're doing. These aren't things to take lightly, and if they involve a certain amount of sacrifice here and there, well, that's just the way it is, and it's a small price to pay.

I haven't been on a night out in Cardiff since 2012. The last time I did, it was with Lyds; we'd been to a wedding, and inevitably we came across someone who'd had too much to drink and who wanted to pick a fight, probably just to prove to his mates what a hard man he was.

On another occasion, I was on a stag night and we were in a pub. There was a group of guys there who wanted to chat, and I was being friendly to them, but then it was time for us to leave and to go on to the next venue. One of the men I'd been talking to became aggressive and started manhandling me in an attempt to get me to stay, and I had to grab his hands and yank them off me so I could leave.

It doesn't take much for these kinds of situation to spiral out of control, and then suddenly you're dealing with negative headlines and distractions, which neither the team nor you need.

Take the case of the England cricketer Ben Stokes, who was charged with affray following a fight outside a Bristol nightclub. He was acquitted, but not before he'd missed an Ashes series and lost a sponsorship deal, and following his acquittal he was fined for bringing the game into disrepute.

Now I don't know him from a bar of soap, I've got no axe to grind with him personally and I mention his case for one reason only: that it could all have been avoided if he hadn't put himself there in the first place. Don't give people the opportunity to make you look bad.

People remember you and judge you as they see you. It doesn't matter what kind of day you're having; the professional thing to do is to smile and make time for people. What's a few seconds for you might mean a whole lot to them. As Ben always reminds me, an autograph or a selfie might be my 100th of the day, but for them it's their first. That's why I always made time for auto-graphs; they don't take up much time and they mean a lot to the person receiving them.

Having been on the other side of the fence, trust me, you remember these things. In the summer of 1999, Mum and Dad took us to Copenhagen. Spurs had won the League Cup a few months before with a 1–0 victory over Leicester City, and Allan Nielsen had scored the winning goal.

In my 10-year-old mind, the logic was clear. Nielsen was Danish, we were in Denmark, therefore we were definitely going to see him. Dad tried to explain that Denmark was a big place with millions of people, so we weren't going to see Allan Nielsen.

But one day, in the Tivoli Gardens, there he was! I plucked up the courage to go over and ask him for an autograph, and to this day I remember how nice he was: asking my name, where I was from, that kind of stuff. I was so thrilled that Mum laminated the piece of paper with his autograph, and for years it was my pride and joy. So when a kid asks for my autograph, I always remember that I could be their Allan Nielsen.

As Alan Phillips said to me: 'People are looking at you and they're dreaming, aren't they? When they look at you, these people, when they see you, they're seeing their dreams.' That was my responsibility as a professional: to be worthy of their dreams.

3

EDEN PARK

36.8750°S, 174.7448°E

**Saturday, 15 October 2011. Wales v France,
World Cup semi-final**

*Come on, son. Come and have a go if you think you're hard
enough.*

*Vincent Clerc comes flying onto the pop pass. I line him up
perfectly, driving up and forward with all the force I can muster
as I hit him. I absolutely unload on him. But he's two stone
lighter than me, so suddenly he's up in the air and his body's
twisting beyond the horizontal.*

*So I let go. Clerc hits the deck and I'm on him again, compet-
ing for the ball and ripping it from him. That's an awesome
tackle, I'm thinking. I've melted him there. That one's going on
my all-time highlight reel for sure.*

*The next thing I know, there's a French fist in my face, and
another one, and the Welsh lads are hauling me up and away
while the French forwards are still trying to use me as a
punchbag.*

Alain Rolland blows his whistle and beckons me over. I

reckon it's a safety thing. I don't even think it's a penalty, let alone a yellow card.

Rolland reaches into his pocket and pulls out the red card.

Monday, 9 May. 'I'm calling to see if you'd like to be captain against the Barbarians.'

I'm speechless. I don't know what to say.

Actually, that's not quite true. I do know what to say, but I don't think Gats would like to hear it. *I hate captaincy.* That's what I'm thinking. *I hate captaincy. I don't want to do it. I'm just 22 years of age. I've only started 10 games for Wales. I'm one of the quieter members of the squad. I'm not given to rousing speeches. Off the top of my head, I can think of half a dozen guys who'd be better at it than me, who have the experience and the personality to do it: Alun Wyn Jones, Stephen Jones, Bomb (Adam Jones), Gethin, Shane, Phillsy (Mike Phillips).*

I'm standing in the front room of my house. I glance at the mirror above the fireplace. I look as stunned as I feel. I never expected this, not in a month of Sundays.

On the other end of the phone, Gats is silent, waiting for me to answer.

Why me? He must see something in me. Buggered if I know what it is, though. But he's a smart coach and a smart guy, and I trust him, so whatever it is, he must genuinely believe in it.

And it's an honour, of course it is. You don't turn down selection for your country, do you? So why would you turn down the captaincy? The only bigger honour than the first is the second. You take each one and do it to the best of your ability.

'Yes, of course,' I say. 'I'd love to do it.'

'Great. There's a press conference at the Millennium in half an hour.'

Flippin' heck. I go upstairs three steps at a time, grab a Welsh Rugby Union polo shirt, slip on some tracksuit bottoms and trainers, and rush out of the door, phone crooked in my neck as I ring first Rach and then Dad.

They both ask me the same question: 'Do you *want* to do it?'

And I give them both the same answer. 'I have to.'

All the way to the stadium, driving with a calmness I don't feel, two words chase each other through my head. *Wales captain. Wales captain. Wales captain.*

In Portugal with Rach. So much for a week of relaxation and switching off. I'm in the gym twice a day, and in the small hours I'm wide awake, making notes about what to say and do.

'Please just switch off,' Rach says.

I can't. I'm worrying about anything and everything.

It's only for this match, I tell myself. *It's only because Gats wants to rest Smiler – Matthew Rees, the regular captain. Maybe Gats is doing it to get me out of my shell a bit, the same way he asked me to stand up in front of the boys and talk about defence and the contact area before the Italy match a couple of months ago. Maybe that's why he hasn't given it to one of the more experienced boys like Stephen or Alun Wyn. Yeah, that makes sense. He wants me to speak up a bit more, take more of an active role once Smiler's back. I'll do it this once and then never again.*

When it's announced that Gavin Henson will be playing for us – his first match in a Wales shirt for two years, even though he's currently not attached to a club – I almost weep with joy. All the media coverage will be about his return rather than my captaincy. Gavin's a hundred times more box office than I'll ever be, and that suits me fine.

Sergio Parisse is captaining the Barbarians. He's a class player, and we know we have to get to him early and often. 'Put the heat on him,' Shaun Edwards tells us.

'Shall we have a call for that?' says Josh Turnbull.

Shaun looks at him like he's mad. 'Get up and f***ing twat him. That's the call.'

Saturday, 4 June. One thing's totally clear in my mind: we cannot, must not, dare not lose to the Barbarians. It's not that they don't have good players, because they have some great ones: Doug Howlett on the wing, Carl Hayman at prop, and a back row I know well: van Niekerk, Martyn and Parisse.

It's that they won't be taking it seriously, because that's the whole ethos of the Barbarians. Five-star hotel, all expenses paid, out on the piss day and night, and five grand at the end of it.

That's why I'll never play for them, because for someone like me it's a lose-lose proposition. If I go with tradition and drink a lot when I so rarely drink, I'll play terribly and it will be bad for my reputation. If I prepare well, as I do for every match I play, everyone will think I'm a shit bloke and boring. The

Barbarians are a great tradition and a longstanding part of rugby, but they're not for me and I'm not for them.

So I just can't even begin to conceive that my first match – my only match, hopefully – as captain is going to be a defeat. I want not just to beat the Barbarians but to humiliate them, to show that in this day and age you need to take international rugby seriously.

I've had enough of the team playing well but coming up a bit short, which has happened all too often in the past couple of seasons, and I've also had enough of people accepting that a little too easily. With the changing of the guard has to come a change in attitude too. After this match there are only three more warm-up matches before the World Cup. If we fancy ourselves to do well in the World Cup, and we do, we have to win this one.

We don't.

Oh, we should do. We're nine points up with nine minutes to go, and from a position like that we ought to be home and hosed. Just keep the ball tight and work it through the phases, running down the clock as we do so. But we're not ruthless enough. Mathieu Bastareaud scores a try to bring them to within a score, and then with a minute to go they run it from deep, Willie Mason offloads out of the tackle to Isa Nacewa, and Nacewa beats four players in a 65-metre run to touch down. The conversion makes it 31–28 to them, and that's that.

I try to rationalise it. *They were a good team, they had nothing to lose. We were missing a few players. That's how it goes.* But whichever way I look at it, we shouldn't have lost.

July. Spala, Poland. You can't win a match you've just lost, but you can win the next one. The only way to atone for the Barbarians defeat is to do well at the World Cup. The only way to do well at the World Cup is to be the fittest team there. The only way to be the fittest team at the World Cup is to push ourselves further than ever before.

Hence Spala.

It was built in the 1950s and still looks like the kind of place where they'd have trained Soviet cosmonauts. It's spartan, in every way. No frills, no fripperies, no distractions. No TV, no PlayStation or Xbox, and no alcohol, not for anybody; drier than a backwoods county in the Bible Belt of the Deep South. Oak forests all around, swaddling us away from the outside world.

You're hard men who've lived soft lives, they tell us. Not any more, not while you're here at any rate. You're going to push yourselves and each other harder and harder, to be quicker and stronger and more durable than you ever thought possible; a hundred and fifty per cent harder than ever before, our strength and conditioning coach Adam Beard says. Take the maximum you've known and add on another half of that again.

This is not a joke. This is not a figure of speech. A hundred and fifty per cent. Add on another half again.

And the pain. Always the pain. We hurt. We hurt together.

We're split into three groups: front five, back row and half-backs, centres and back three. We have three hour-long sessions a day. The sessions are staggered, so we wait our turn while the group before us is being beasted. We wait in silence, readying ourselves for the pain. As we go out to start a session, we pass the guys before us coming back in. They have the glassy-eyed look of a convicts' road gang. They're all dripping with sweat. Quite a few are splattered with vomit.

Weight vests on, stiff with the sweat of whoever used them last. Standing in a sandpit lifting heavy bags from ground to head and back. Pushing weighted sleds. Tyre flips. Bear crawls. Down and up, sprint, down and up, sprint.

Throw up? Good. Better out than in. Keep going. Trying to suck in the air. Shattered. Don't show it. Don't put your hands on your knees. That's Rule One. Never put your hands on your knees.

Thank God that's over.

'One more circuit.'

Wrestling, one-on-one with Jonathan Thomas. He's three inches taller and a stone and a half heavier than me. Money passing between Gats and Rob Howley as they watch. 'A tenner says JT.' I look up long enough to snarl at them, which is exactly the response they want.

Tug-of-war, one-on-one with Bradley Davies: six inches taller, three stone heavier, and a real athlete. Gats doesn't care. 'Fancy yourself up there with McCaw, Warby? Bradley's making you his bitch.'

I set myself and pull harder. Every muscle screaming in agony. I can take it.

The management watching us like hawks the whole time. Who's going to crack? Who's going to break? Who's going to whinge? Do any of those and you aren't going to the World Cup. You keep going because the next guy does, and the next guy keeps going because you do. If you break that chain then you have no place here.

Into the cryotherapy chambers. Shorts, socks, gloves, face mask, headband and wooden clogs. The first chamber is at -50°C, but that's just a warm-up, if you like, for the second chamber. The second chamber is -150°C: a whiteout where you can't see the guy standing right next to you, where you keep talking and moving for fear that if you don't you'll just stop and die. Even the tiniest drop of sweat left over stings as it freezes hard on your skin.

This kind of cold is a living thing: something that scours, something that sears. It's not just that it helps repair damaged tissues quicker, allowing us to train harder. It's a mental thing too, a purging. The cold strips away everything but the essentials. Cleanse yourself. Punish yourself. You want to win? This is what it takes.

This is the kind of thing that bonds teams together, so that in the last few minutes of a tight match you can look at each other and know what everyone's thinking without needing to say it.

Remember Spala.

Remember Spala, and know that you have what it takes to close out the win. We've lost too many of those kind of matches. Not anymore.

Remember Spala.

Smiler's suffering from a neck injury, so I keep the captaincy for the two warm-up matches against England in August, first at Twickenham, then a week later in Cardiff.

Andy helps me develop a leadership compass: four attributes that will make me a better captain.

- Professional attitude
- Positive attitude
- My own performance, and leading by example
- Develop personal relationships with the players

The first three come easily to me, the fourth less so, simply because I'm quite introverted and shy. Work on that one more than the others, Andy says. Sometimes you have to work on your weaknesses rather than your strengths, at least to get them to the point where they're no longer a weakness.

Saturday, 6 August. Twickenham. I write reams and reams on the hotel notepad before the first England match, pacing up and down the room, practising what I'm going to say. But when it comes to giving the team talk, it all comes out as just a bunch of mumbled irrelevant crap. It would be bad enough as it is, but much worse that I've spent so much time and energy on it for so little reward.

We lose the match 23–19, though the result pales into insignificance compared with the horrific injury that Morgan Stoddart suffers early in the second half. He wasn't even supposed to be on the pitch so soon, but Stephen had pulled up with a calf injury in the warm-up, forcing us to switch Rhys Priestland to 10 and bring Morgan in at 15.

Morgan's tackled from behind by Delon Armitage, and his left leg goes two different ways at once. Danny Care, fair play to him, instantly sees the trouble Morgan's in and frantically calls the ref to blow up so Morgan can get treatment. He's snapped both his tibia and fibula, and he's screaming in pain. It's a break so horrific that they don't even show it on the TV replay, and it's a reminder to everyone that there but for the grace of God go us all. It wasn't a foul or a dirty tackle, just a tragic accident.

Morgan's out of the World Cup, that much is immediately obvious. What we don't know at the time is that he'll never play for Wales again.

Saturday, 13 August. Millennium. I don't use any notes or prepare a speech this time. I just speak off the cuff and from the heart. I keep it simple. What are the three things we need to win this game? Discipline, work rate, belief. Nothing special, nothing Churchillian. It's England at the Millennium. That's enough in itself.

We're level pegging at half-time, 6–6, and in the second half we stretch away to win 19–9. It's the seventh time I've played an England representative side – Under-16s, Under-18s, Under-19s, Under-20s, in the Six Nations earlier this year and at Twickenham last week – and the first time I've ever beaten them.

God, it feels sweet. It's not that I hate England – how can I, when my dad's English? – and I certainly don't have that mentality typical of some Welsh people that beating England is the be-all and end-all of Welsh rugby. But when you've only ever known defeat against a side and you finally get one over on them, it means more and tastes better than just your average common or garden victory.

'Smiler's out.'

'What do you mean, Smiler's out?'

'His neck injury's worse than we thought. We'd reckoned he could get through the World Cup and have surgery when the tournament's over, but there's no chance of that now. In Poland there were times when he couldn't sleep for the pain. Losing feeling in his hands, that kind of stuff. Really struggling. He needs half a disc removed, and he's going under the knife in Bristol any day now.'

Poor Smiler. He must be gutted. Every player dreams of playing in the World Cup. But I know what's coming.

'So,' Gats says, 'we'd like you to carry on as skipper on a permanent basis. To the World Cup, and beyond.'

Smiler rings me. He's still on the ward after his operation.

'Gats says you're not sure about taking the captaincy,' he says.

'Yeah. I just feel it's too early for me. I don't captain the Blues, and I'm still quite new in the national set-up.'

'Well, that's one of the reasons Gats wants you. He's looking long-term, for the next few seasons rather than the next few matches, just like the All Blacks have done with McCaw. And for what it's worth I think you'll do a great job. You're guaranteed a starting spot, you'll get a lot of help from the senior boys like Gethin and Alun Wyn, and most of all everybody in the squad respects you and likes you.'

Maybe, I think, but I know quite a few of the senior players disagree with my selection as captain. No one says anything bad to my face, but I can still tell. I guess that if I had 60 or 70 caps and fancied my chances as captain, and then someone with a quarter of that number was suddenly catapulted over the top of me into the hot seat, I'd probably feel the same way too. Knowing that there's disapproval out there makes me feel as though I'm walking round with a sign hanging from my

neck and a huge weight on my shoulders, both of them drag-
ging me down when I should be standing tall and proud.

'Listen,' Smiler continues. 'When I was first offered the role I wasn't sure either, even though I'd already played for the Lions. Anyone with any sense doubts themselves. But I got great support and felt more comfortable with every game that passed. You'll find the same. Trust me. Opportunities like this don't come round too often, and if you turn it down you'll kick yourself.'

I really appreciate Smiler's call and I tell Gats I'll do it, but deep down I'm still not sure. And I'm so immature in some ways that I can't bring myself to front up and tell Gats my worries, even though I see him every day at training. I use Andy as an intermediary, which is chicken of me but at least gives me the chance to talk through things with him first.

'I hate captaincy,' I say. 'It's a strong word, but it's the right one. I hate it.'

'OK,' Andy replies. 'What don't you like about it?'

'I hate having a room on my own. I like having someone to bounce off.'

'I'm sure we can change that. What else?'

'I hate doing press.' Not because I dislike the journalists personally – quite the opposite, they're mostly good guys who know their rugby – but because all that press stuff gets in the way of everything else. The other day I had to miss lunch to do the press conference, but I couldn't afford not to eat, so I got a plate of turkey, potatoes and vegetables, put it in a blender, added water and drank it like a protein shake. And yes, it was every bit as rank as it sounds.

Or I might have to miss the analysis sessions, which means I have to catch up on the calls and the moves everyone else knows perfectly, and then I risk being the one who messes it up. I especially hate live interviews, because they always want you there 20 minutes early and so you're kicking your heels all that time for what ends up being a 90-second piece.

'OK,' says Andy. 'Let's ask that you do press once a week, no more. What else?'

'Sponsorship appearances.'

'What about them?'

'There are too many.'

'Then let's delegate them among the boys.'

It sounds so simple, because it is, but until Andy goes through all this with me I don't realise that captaincy, like everything, is give and take. Very few things are set in stone, and there's almost always room for discussion. When we take my concerns to Gats, he's fine with all of them.

But even so, he senses that I'm still unsure.

'Have a look at this,' he says.

It's a clip from our victory over England at the Millennium. I tackle Mark Cueto, then immediately jump back up and take my position in the defensive line. Josh Turnbull competes at the ruck and wins the penalty. Immediately I march to the ruck, punching the air, pulling Josh to his feet and slapping his back, geeing everybody up.

Gats pauses the clip. 'That's leadership,' he says simply.

Now I'm beginning to get it. I smile and begin to walk away.

'Sam,' he calls out. I turn. He's pointing to my new spon-sored Range Rover. 'If you still don't want to be captain, your profile won't be as high and Land Rover might take that nice car off you.'

He smirks. I laugh. He's got a point.

In his book *The Captain Class*, Sam Walker, former global sports editor at the *Wall Street Journal*, identifies seven traits that elite captains demonstrate. What Gats has just shown me is an example of one of them: 'motivates others with passionate nonverbal displays'.

The others are:

- extreme doggedness and focus in competition
- aggressive play that tests the limits of the rules
- a willingness to do thankless jobs in the shadows
- a low-key, practical and democratic communication style
- strong convictions and the courage to stand apart
- ironclad emotional control

As descriptions of both my style of play and my personality, all seven seem pretty much spot on.

Friday, 2 September. We land in Wellington. Including the time difference, it's two days since we left home.

We go for a walk to help ease the stiffness after so long in an aeroplane. Look, someone says, there's a bar up ahead. Let's go get a drink.

The bar is called Mermaids. There are a few half-dressed women in there, and a pole on a stage, but we're all a bit jetlagged and zonked so we don't really twig what's going on.

We think it's just a mildly risqué place. Most of us order coffee. A couple of the boys have a beer.

Then we see it. A huge, illuminated neon arrow pointing up the stairs, and beneath it in equally huge illuminated letters the word 'SEX'.

We're in a brothel.

We finish up our drinks a lot quicker than we started them and get the hell out. It's only a couple of weeks since England made headlines for all the wrong reasons with their dwarf-tossing in a Queenstown bar, and if there'd been someone around with a camera we could easily have been in the same position, spending days dealing with the fallout and the negative publicity rather than concentrating on preparing ourselves for the tournament.

It was an innocent mistake, but try telling that to the press pack and the social media hordes. We've dodged a bullet there, and we know it. That's one of the advantages of not being a high-profile team like England: we can fly under the radar a little. I hope we can stay there for a while.

It's my first time in New Zealand. When Gats first came over to be interviewed for the Wales job, the WRU chief executive Roger Lewis took him on a helicopter trip over South Wales. Villages and towns dotted with rugby pitches, fields and hillsides lush with rain, valleys and the mountainous beauty of the Brecon Beacons – Lewis knew just what he was doing.

'It looks like New Zealand,' Gats said.

It does. And now I'm here, I see that the reverse is obviously true too – that New Zealand looks like Wales. The similarity doesn't stop there. Both countries have got small, rugby-mad populations: just over three million for us, just under five million for them. England, France, South Africa, Australia and the rest of the big names here – their populations are too big, their range of other sports too large, for rugby to capture the soul of the nation in the way that it does us and New Zealand.

I feel right at home.

In Wales, the most celebrated position on the field is number 10, the fly-half. Think of the men who've played there: Cliff Morgan, Barry John, Phil Bennett, Jonathan Davies, Neil Jenkins, Stephen Jones.

New Zealand have produced their share of excellent fly-halves too, but for them the sacred number isn't 10. It's 7. Before Richie McCaw was Josh Kronfeld, before Kronfeld was Michael Jones, and before Jones was Graham Mourie. To be playing 7 in New Zealand, even if you're not playing for New Zealand, is to take on a precious mantle.

Gats and I are in a press conference before our first pool match against South Africa. 'There are three definite world-class players at the breakdown in this tournament,' Gats says. 'David Pocock, Richie McCaw and Heinrich Brüssow. I'd rate the guy next to me in that category as well. A lot of people haven't seen Sam Warburton play, but he'll create an impact in this tournament. He wins man of the match more often than not, and you'll find out why on Sunday.'

Bloody hell, I think. *No pressure, Gats.*

Sunday, 11 September. You never want the hardest game in the group first up, because if you lose, then every game after that becomes a must-win. Even if those must-win games are ones you should win, it still alters the equation a little bit. But we didn't choose the schedule and we can't alter it, so there's no point complaining. Crack on. Game on.

I lead the boys out in Wellington. At 22 years and 341 days old, I'm the youngest World Cup captain ever. I'm up against a seriously talented back row – Brüssow, Schalk Burger and Pierre Spies – but I feel invincible, and I play like it too. This is the best international match I've played so far, and only perhaps one or two more in the future will match it.

I'm everywhere. I make 23 tackles, almost a quarter of the team's entire total. I secure six turnovers. I'm faster to every breakdown than the AA could dream of. No matter how quick the Boks are, I'm quicker, and it really pisses them off. As the game wears on I can hear them shouting more and more at each breakdown: 'Smash him. Get him off the ball!'

They try and clear me out by fair means or foul. I cop a massive blow to my head and can hardly stand up for a moment or two while the world spins, but I'm there at the next breakdown, and the next one, and the next one after that.

I win man of the match. And we lose the game. Only by a point, 17–16, but a loss is a loss. It doesn't matter how well I played, because we lost. But it does matter how well I captain, because I make one mistake that may have a big effect on the result.

It's the 14th minute. Hooky – James Hook – kicks a penalty so high that it passes over the top of the upright. From where I'm standing, it's hard to tell whether it's just in or just out. The assistant referees watch the ball in flight, look at each other and keep their flags down: no score. The referee, Wayne Barnes, agrees.

Even though both Hooky and Jenks think it's gone over – Hooky's so confident that he starts running back to the half-way line for the kick-off – I don't think of questioning it. The moment comes and goes so quickly that I'm almost not aware of it. I should question it, but I don't. It's just not me, to confront something like that. Ironic that I'm happy to confront enormous Springbok forwards all day but not ask a simple question of the officials, but there you go. I've never been the kind of person to complain in restaurants or make a fuss in public, and that feeds through into this.

It might not make a difference, of course. The officials might decide after looking at a replay that there's no reason to change their minds; and even if they do, it's so early in the game that there's plenty of time for South Africa to come back, and maybe they'd change their tactics if they were two points down rather than a point up. Rugby's rarely as simple as saying that a single incident would leave the rest of the match unaltered.

In years to come, this respect for referees and their decisions will become one of my biggest strengths. But right now it feels like a huge weakness, and even though I can't change what's happened, I resolve that if it ever occurs in the future I won't make the same mistake again.

Losing to South Africa means that, assuming we both win all our other pool matches, we'll come second in the group and face the winner of Pool C in the quarters. That's almost certain to be Australia, whose toughest match in that pool is against Ireland. We've only won one of our last six games against the Wallabies. You can say all you like about having to play the good teams sooner or later, but Australia in the quarters would be a big ask.

The Irish turn them over 15–6.

Suddenly, all the permutations are flipped 180 degrees. Now it's almost certain that we'd play Ireland in the quarters, which is a far easier prospect. We know Ireland's game so well, we beat them in the Six Nations, and we reckon we've more than got the measure of them.

We're looking at a semi-final here, I think, as long as we don't screw it up.

Sunday, 18 September. Hamilton. We almost do screw it up. We're 10–6 down to Samoa at half-time, and if we lose this that's zero points from two games and we're almost certainly on an early flight home.

I don't know what to say to the boys in the dressing room, but Shane Williams does. He gives us all the most almighty bollocking. 'There's no way we're going to lose this,' he yells, 'not after everything we've been through.'

Remember Spala.

Samoa are without doubt the dirtiest team I've played against; at one point I get someone's heel in my face as I'm lying on the floor, and it's not an accident. Stung by the thought of going home, we take it to them physically. We pluck it fast off lineouts, Jamie runs over Seilala Mapusua in the 12 channel, we work it through the biggest forwards until there's space out wide and we can spread it. They don't score a point in the second half, and we run out winners 17–6. It's not pretty, but the result's all that matters. Very few teams ever go through tournaments playing brilliantly all the time and swatting aside every opponent.

Now we know we'll be in the quarters, because with the best will in the world we're not going to lose either of our remaining matches to Namibia or Fiji.

Monday, 26 September. New Plymouth. There's a moment against Namibia which means a lot to me, even though no one in the stands and few people on the pitch even notice. We have a penalty, and I tell Stephen to go for the three points rather than kick to the corner and go for a lineout within range of their tryline.

I know some of the boys will think this is me being too conservative, and that I should be being ruthless against a team who are never really going to trouble us – we'll end up beating them 81–7 – but Stephen quiets any dissent.

'Warby, you're our captain,' he says. 'Whatever you say, we're doing.'

From someone with more than 100 caps, that's an endorsement I appreciate.

Sunday, 2 October. Hamilton. On the bus back from the Fiji game, as pleased with the zero points we conceded as the 66 we scored, I'm looking out of the window when I get a sudden and rather weird rush of feeling: a wave of positivity and excitement. We're going to do something here. We're going to do something special.

Saturday, 8 October. It's wet and windy in Wellington – when is it not? – so at least we've got conditions that wouldn't be out of place in either Cardiff or Dublin. Everyone's talking about the back rows, because whenever we play Ireland it seems to be a massive cock-off as to who's got the best.

Theirs is pretty good – Stephen Ferris, Sean O'Brien and Jamie Heaslip – but I reckon that Lyds, Toby Faletau and I have got the measure of them. Go low, Shaun says before the start. Go low at them, get their big men to the ground, chop tackle them all day long. Lyds tackles, I jackal. That's how we'll win our battles.

We're ahead within three minutes. We run what we call 'pattern' and everyone else calls 'Warrenball', Jamie doing his usual battering-ram impression up the middle and working the phases from that to put Shane over in the corner. Rhys Priestland nails a very difficult kick, given the conditions, and we're seven points up almost before we've started.

We're never headed, even though Ireland do bring it back to 10–10 just after half-time. It's a proper old-school Test match, intense and brutal, full of blood and thunder. They spend long periods attacking, but we just stand firm and soak it up, a red line spread across the pitch. When one team attacks and attacks without the scores to show for it, their self-belief inevitably starts to ebb away.

That's what happens here. By the time we get to the last quarter, we know we've got them. They're only five points behind, but they look tired and under the cosh; and when Foxy (Jonathan Davies, whose parents own a pub called The Fox and Hounds) scores we know it's all over. The Welsh fans spend the last 15 minutes singing 'Delilah' over and over.

'The biggest regret of my career,' Brian O'Driscoll will call this match when he retires in three years' time. They obviously fancied their chances as much as we fancied ours, and either of us would back ourselves to win the semi against a France side so lacklustre that they lost twice in the pool stages and have effectively sacked their coach mid-tournament. But it's Ireland who are going home and we who've got two more weeks here (even if we lose the semi, there's the third-place play-off two days before the final).

Mum and Dad book themselves flights out for the semi-final.

Wednesday, 12 October. I'm walking back to the hotel when a Kiwi bloke comes up and starts telling me how well I'm playing and what a great 7 I am. I thank him, but since this kind of stuff really embarrasses me I try to change the subject.

'What about McCaw?' I say. 'He's pretty good, to say the least.'

'Maybe.'

'Maybe? Why maybe?'

'He hasn't won the World Cup yet.'

I'm like, you what? But he's being deadly serious. George Smith, Phil Waugh, Neil Back, François Pienaar: those guys won World Cups, he says. McCaw can't count himself as being up there with them until he does the same.

That's how high the Kiwis set the bar for success. I can't work out whether it's inspiring or intimidating. Probably a bit of both.

Andy has come on tour with us. It was a choice between him and a third video analyst, and it went to a vote. The video boys were gutted, because it increased their workload by a third. But the fact that the majority of the boys voted for Andy shows how influential he is, even though – or perhaps especially because – so much of his work is confidential. Sometimes the coaches tell him that they never actually see him doing anything, and each time he just smiles and replies, 'That shows I'm doing my job.'

The identity statement I've been working on with him has changed. Before, it was 'I want to be the world's best 7.' That's no longer an aspiration; it's a fact. 'I am the world's best 7.' A big call, especially given the rare strength in depth of 7s at this competition, but over the five games of the tournament so far I honestly believe I've played better than any of my rivals.

Friday, 14 October. Gats and I go and see Alain Rolland, who'll be refereeing the semi-final tomorrow. (He's Irish, despite the French-sounding name.)

'I've got nothing, really,' Rolland says, 'so you guys crack on.'

That's a bit strange, I think. Refs usually have a couple of things they want to chat about, especially before a game as big as this; things they've seen in previous rounds, things they're going to be keeping a close eye on.

But Rolland has none of that. He's not as friendly as I thought he'd be; blasé, in fact. It's almost like he doesn't want to be here.

Saturday, 15 October. Semi-final day. I go to Andy's room, ready for our usual pre-match chat reinforcing the positives, but I'm hardly through the door when I realise something.

I'm ready.

I don't need the chat, not today. It's the first time that's ever happened. I'm so perfectly prepared that I don't need anything other than what I've already done. I don't feel in the slightest bit nervous or apprehensive. Quite the opposite, in fact. I feel like a superhero, so full of confidence that it's practically bursting out of me. I want to play right now, this minute.

We're going to win. I don't just think that or hope that; I know it. We're going to win. We're going to beat France, and we're going to be in the World Cup Final.

I walk out of that room feeling ten feet tall.

Huddling in the changing-room with the boys.

'The bravest team wins,' I say. 'We've got to give things a go. If your gut says go for something, then do it. Don't go into your shell. Winners don't wait for chances – they take them. They *make* them. Let's not die wondering.'

History so close I can practically taste it. No team outside the big five – Australia, England, France, New Zealand and South Africa – have ever reached a World Cup Final. We'd be the first. Back home in Cardiff the Millennium is full, a packed breakfast time crowd watching us live on the big screens there. The Welsh flag is flying over 10 Downing Street. Even most Kiwis seem to be backing us – they like our attitude, they like the way we play – though equally they reckon we'd be a bigger threat than France in the final.

We are 9 kg a man heavier in the scrum. Let's use it.

William Servat runs hard. Toby tackles him and I jackal, slowing the ball down and allowing our defence to get back in position. Don't let them run the ball in broken field play, not the French of all people. Dimitri Yachvili chips through and Pence knocks on into touch. Slippery ball, nervous hands.

Imanol Harinordoquy runs at me, and I knock him back. I tackle Thierry Dusautoir, one openside on the other. Damn, I feel strong. Rolland pings Dusautoir for offside at a ruck and we have the penalty. It's out near the touchline, but Hooky says he can get it – and he does, curling it in beautifully to make it 3–0. First blood.

Nine minutes gone. Bomb signals to the bench. He's done his calf and can't continue. That's a huge blow – the tighthead is the cornerstone of the scrum, and Bomb's got the better of everyone he's played against. Of all the people we don't want to lose early doors, he's right up there. But it's happened, so there's no point worrying or complaining about it. Crack on.

Paul James's first scrum as Bomb's replacement is a good one; down go the French, and it's another penalty to us. It's easier than the first one, but Hooky's standing foot slips as he connects and the ball's pushed wide. Hooky checks the studs on his left boot.

On the bench, Bomb has his head in his hands. When he looks up, his eyes are red with tears.

The first 15 minutes are all ours: more than two-thirds territory and 50 per cent more kicking metres than them. Phillsy pops it to me short and I make good ground through the defence, with Gethin and Alun Wyn flying in behind me. We work it wide. Shane switches with Jamie, but the pass is too high and Foxy knocks on. We're all over them, absolutely all over them.

Seventeen minutes gone. They have a lineout just inside our half. I know they often use a move from the tail of lineouts like this, with their scrum-half peeling round and the blindside winger coming in at pace.

'At every set piece,' Steve Williams once told me back in Whitchurch, 'take an extra couple of seconds, just to have a look. What are the backline doing? What's their body language? Who's switched off, so you know they're not getting the call, and who's switched on? What can you get a read on?'

I take those couple of seconds now.

There. Vincent Clerc, their blindside winger, is setting himself like a sprinter: hitching up his shorts, crouching low, looking left and right. Either he's going to be running decoy or he's having it. Either way, he's mine. I'm the tail gunner at the back of the lineout, so it's my job to take the first threat to the backline.

In a similar situation during the Ireland match I made a mistake, and I know the French analysts will have picked up on it. If they think I'm a weakness, bring it on. I'm not making the same mistake twice. If Clerc comes down my channel, I'll give him something to think about.

The French put six men in their lineout and throw to Julien Bonnaire in the middle. We've got no lifting pod at the back, so we can easily get stuck in to the maul. We all know our roles. 'I've got 9!' Lyds shouts. If Yachvili snipes round the side, Lyds will chop him. I don't need to worry about Yachvili. I go one more out, and now my options are down from three to two: either Parra at 10 or Clerc coming in from 14.

Come on, son. Come and have a go if you think you're hard enough.

Clerc comes flying onto the pop pass. I line him up perfectly, driving up and forward with all the force I can muster as I hit him. I absolutely unload on him. I hit him as hard as I would one of their locks or props, because you can't go into a tackle half-heartedly. But Clerc's two stone lighter than me, so suddenly he's up in the air and his body's twisting beyond the horizontal. I've got not just weight and strength on my side but momentum too, as he slows down just before impact. If I keep holding on his legs will go higher still, I'll drill him head first into the ground, Lyds and Toby will be coming in right behind me, and all that could get very ugly, very fast, and mean a nasty injury for the lad.

All this is going through my head in the blink of an eye.

So I let go. Clerc hits the deck and I'm on him again, competing for the ball and ripping it from him. *That's an awesome tackle*, I'm thinking. *I've melted him there. That one's going on my all-time highlight reel for sure.*

The next thing I know, there's a French fist in my face, and another one, and the Welsh lads are hauling me up and away while the French forwards are still trying to use me as a punch-bag. At least they're not grabbing my bollocks.

I honestly don't know what the fuss is about. I did almost identical tackles twice in the quarters, one on Ronan O'Gara and the other on Stephen Ferris, and neither one caused a problem. Clerc's lying on the ground, holding his head and writhing around a bit as the physios crouch over him; he's making a meal of it, I reckon, in a rather French way.

Rolland blows his whistle and beckons me over. I reckon it's a safety thing. He'll remind me that it's the tackler's responsibility to bring the tackled player to earth safely, and I'll say it's precisely because I had Clerc's safety in mind that I let go to stop him being hurt. I honestly can't see how it can be any more than that. I don't even think it's a penalty, let alone a yellow card.

Rolland reaches into his pocket and pulls out the red card. With his right hand, he holds it high above his head, with his left he points me to the touchline.

For a split second my mind goes blank, just unable to compute what I'm seeing. Then a single thought goes through my head. *Don't complain.* Don't argue, don't remonstrate, don't protest. I've seen enough footballers do that, and I really hate it. It's disrespectful and it's pointless, as the referee's never going to change his mind. Just walk off. No matter how unfair it seems, button it and walk off.

That's just what I do. A camera follows me all the way. *Don't swear*, I'm thinking. I remember an Under-20s match against Japan in Swansea three years before when I'd been sinbinned for an accidental high tackle. The match was shown on S4C, and there I was caught on camera effing and jeffing like a petulant child. My mum gave me a right clip for that, and deservedly so. And that's all I can think right now: if I use even a single curse word, it'll be shown all around the world and my mum – who's in the stands today – will give me another clip.

It's like a bad dream. I sit heavily down onto the bench, the camera still in my face, and think of all the things I should have done before leaving the pitch: got the boys in, handed the captaincy to Alun Wyn, told them all that this is a real test of character and let's prove all the doubters wrong. I didn't do any of that. I should have done. I should have stepped out of my personal bubble and looked at the bigger picture.

'What are you doing?' Jenks says.

'I'm off, mate.'

'For that? That's ridiculous. Anyway, get a coat on you. Keep warm anyway. It's only ten minutes.'

'Mate, it's not yellow. It's red.'

Jenks goes nuts, kicking the air, raging at the assistant referee. In the ITV commentary box, though obviously I don't know this until later, Nick Mullins and Michael Owen both think the same thing, that I've got a yellow, and it's a few seconds before the red card logo comes up on the screen and you can hear the total disbelief in their voices.

I feel about three inches high. The biggest match of my life, captain of my country in a World Cup semi-final, and I've let everyone down before even a quarter of the match is over. The team, the fans, the country – I've let them all down.

I sit on that bench for the remaining 22 minutes of the half, and it's the longest 22 minutes of my life. I don't say anything, I don't want to storm off down the tunnel in a huff, I don't want to give the cameraman – who's never more than three metres from me all this time – the satisfaction of showing any kind of emotion whatsoever. They keep replaying the tackle on the big screen, and in slow-motion it looks a lot worse than it felt at the time.

After what seems aeons, Rolland blows for half-time and I can go down the tunnel with the rest of the boys. France are 6–3 ahead.

I don't speak at half-time. What can I say? It's up to the others now, and I can't do a damn thing to help them, which is as bad a feeling as being sent off in the first place. I come back out with them for the second half and take up my position on the bench again, a helpless bystander.

That second half is agony. Parra scores another penalty to make it 9–3. With just over 20 minutes left, Phillsy snipes off the side of a ruck, shows and goes between the two French locks and scores near the left-hand corner.

It's 9–8. We're a point down, but we'll be a point up when Stephen nails this conversion – which he will, because for a man of his class it's a sitter. He'd kick this nine times out of ten.

This is that tenth time. It hits the post and bounces out.

A calf strain. A red card. A missed kick. That sense that it's just not our day.

We're still a point down, and that's how it stays for the rest of the match. With six minutes left, Pence has a penalty shot from halfway, and though the kick has the direction it doesn't quite have the distance. In the final moments we work 26 phases, but then Jamie knocks on and it's all over.

The dressing-room's like a morgue. Sometimes when you lose you know there was nothing you could have done; you were beaten fair and square, and that's it. Sometimes you lose by inches and beat yourself up about the tiny things you could have done to change it.

But sometimes, like now, you know it should have been you. We were a better team than them, not just today but through-out the tournament. We trained harder, we rooted for each other more, we committed more.

If we'd had 15 men, we'd have won. If I hadn't got the red card, we'd have won. If Bomb hadn't gone off so early, we'd have won. If Stephen had nailed the conversion, we'd have won.

If, if, if, if.

Phillsy puts his arm around me. 'Don't you dare think that what happened was your fault. It's been an honour to play with you in this tournament.'

One by one, the other boys come up and say similar things. Not a single one of them blames me or has a go. What a gleaming bunch of blokes they are.

I have to say something. I can hardly get the words out.

'I couldn't have asked more of you. Any of you. You couldn't have been braver.'

Then I find an empty toilet cubicle, lock the door behind me and sob my heart out for 15 minutes. Hot, angry tears, letting it all flow out. Tears not just for me but for those I love and respect too. What will my mum and dad be thinking? What will Ben and Holly be thinking? What will Rach be thinking? Or Frank Rees, or Gwyn Morris, or Steve Williams, all of whom taught me and nurtured my talent? They'll be disappointed in me. That's even worse than them being angry with me.

Disappointed. We thought you were better than that, Sam.

When I can trust myself to last a few minutes without crying again, I come out of the toilet and have a shower. I stand in the shower, letting the water beat against the back of my neck as I stare at the floor. I can only imagine the reaction at home to my sending-off. It'll be like what happened to David Beckham after his red card against Argentina in the 1998 World Cup, though obviously on a smaller scale: people blaming me, calling me a dirty player, the man who lost us the World Cup, throwing eggs at my window, maybe even burning an effigy of me on Bonfire Night in a few weeks' time.

Simon Rimmer, the press officer, comes into the dressing-room.

'There's a press conference in ten minutes' time,' he says. 'You don't have to do it if you don't feel up to it.'

It's tempting, to hide myself away and let Gats and maybe Alun Wyn deal with all the questions. But I know this is one presser I really have to do. And actually I want to do it. I don't want to be the kind of guy who shirks the stuff he'd rather avoid. Good blokes are there at shit times; shit blokes are only there at good times. It was my tackle, my card, my dismissal. Own it. Take it on the chin and front up. Besides, if I do this one then it'll nip it in the bud and hopefully I won't have to do any more.

So I tell the press the truth – that there was no malicious intent, that I thought it was a normal tackle, that Clerc's body-weight took control of what happened after I hit him, and that I'm devastated.

When the press conference is over and we've left the room, Shaun Edwards puts his arm around me. 'Welcome to the club,' he says.

I offer a weak smile. In his rugby league days he'd been red-carded for clotheslining Brad Clyde in a Great Britain–Australia Test match.

'The difference is,' Shaun continues, 'I deserved mine and you didn't.'

Numb. Just numb. I've let everyone down, haven't I? Whether or not I deserved the red card, that's what I got. The horror comes in waves, and it's all I can do to ride those waves until they subside a bit and I can begin to think rationally again. I can't remember ever feeling this bad, not about anything. Such an important match in front of so many people … I can hardly believe it. I wish I could say it feels like a dream, but it doesn't. It feels all too real.

I go the hotel bar with Mum and Dad. We all need a drink.

'Where are you guys from?' the barman asks.

'Wales,' my dad says.

'You see the game earlier?'

'We caught some of it, yes.'

'What the hell was their captain thinking? You'd have thought he'd have known better, wouldn't you?'

I look at Mum and Dad. We're all frozen somewhere between disbelief that this is happening and frantically trying not to laugh. I'm half-looking around for a hidden camera somewhere in case this is a TV prank show.

The barman brings us our drinks. A few minutes later, I see one of his colleagues talking urgently to him. They look in our direction. The barman's face drops, and he's out of there like Usain Bolt.

We don't see him again.

Sunday, 16 October. The International Rugby Board (IRB) hearing takes place the afternoon after the match. Five of us, all suited and booted, walk the short distance from the team hotel to the building where the hearing's being held: me, Gats, team manager Alan Phillips, the WRU's lawyer Rhodri Lewis, and Simon Rimmer.

We turn right onto a street full of bars and cafés. Rugby fans are spilling out of pretty much every one of them: men and women in the shirts of their home countries, talking and laughing and drinking. Different languages, different accents, but all connected by their love of the game.

For a moment, I check my stride. This is the very last thing I need, to run a gauntlet of pissed-up fans hurling abuse and telling me what they think of me. I'm just about to look for another way to get to the hearing when I clock that the nearest bunch of fans have seen us. We can't turn around now even if we wanted to; it would look like we were fleeing.

Nothing for it except to hold my head high, keep walking, and not react to anything anyone says on the way past. *It's not far. Block it out. Game head on.*

The nearest bunch of fans start to make a noise, and it's a moment or two before I realise what it is. They're clapping and cheering me. And then the next bunch start to applaud too, and the next bunch, and the next one, a Mexican wave of cheering and appreciation that ripples all the way down the street. It's not just the Welsh fans, it's the French ones and the Aussies and the locals too. Every single one of them letting me know they have my back.

My throat's a lump and my eyes are smarting by the time we make it to the tribunal building. Rugby's got the greatest supporters in the world, it really has.

The photographers inside the building aren't nearly so sympathetic, snapping pictures of me in the lift as though this is a criminal trial.

The hearing itself, conducted by England's Christopher Quinlan, is unsparing. It lasts two hours without a break, and they show the tackle again and again from 13 different angles at real speed and in slow motion. The law in question is 10.4 (j), which states that 'lifting a player from the ground and drop-ping or driving that player into the ground whilst that player's feet are still off the ground such that the player's head and/or upper body come into contact with the ground is dangerous play'.

I tell them that it's for those very reasons that I let go of Clerc, so that I wouldn't be driving him into the ground. They say that I should have kept hold of Clerc and turned him so that the two of us could hit the ground safely, which may be true but is also much easier said than done when things happen so fast.

I accept it was a red card, I say, but I assure them it wasn't deliberate. I'm just not that kind of player. I've had only two yellow cards in the last three seasons, both of them for tech-nical infringements rather than dirty play. Openside is a posi-tion where you have to play right on the edge, more so than any other. Name me another international 7 with a disciplinary record as good as mine.

I tell them that this match is something I've been dreaming about since I was a young lad. This is why I sacrificed so much as a teenager, missing the nights out, the alcohol and all the fun. This is why I trained during every school lunchtime and after school too, why I ran late at night and spent hours in the garage on the multigym.

That, all of that, was geared towards two things: represent-ing Wales, and being the best 7 in the world. Why would I ruin all that by deliberately dump-tackling somebody in such a big match? Haven't I been humiliated enough by having to sit on the sidelines, a camera in my face, watching my side lose a World Cup semi-final?

We leave the room while they consider their verdict.

'Mate, a suspension isn't the worst thing in the world,' Gats says while we wait. 'You could do with the rest.' He thinks a moment, and then deadpans, 'Maybe I should have really laid into you there rather than backed you, to get you as long a lay-off as possible.'

I laugh. Always looking at the big picture, that's Gats.

They call us back in. Quinlan says that the offence has been classified 'mid-range', which usually carries a suspension of at least six weeks, but because of my remorse, good character and disciplinary record, they've halved that. I'm out until 7 November, which means I'll be able to play for the Blues in their Heineken Cup match against Racing Métro on Armistice Day, but I won't be able to play in the third-place play-off against Australia later this week.

It's not just the supporters who are on my side. Lots of former players are too.

François Pienaar says: 'It was a dangerous tackle, yes. A penalty, yes. Never a red card. This is a World Cup semi-final, with all the world watching. You have all the technology at your disposal. Why not go to the video referee or ask your touch judge?'

Phil Bennett says that the ruling may have been 'technically correct, but morally wrong, emotionally wrong, wrong to the bottom of my gut'. And Kobus Wiese says 'the application of the rule must be looked at by the IRB. Take away the red card and cite somebody afterwards to keep the game fair. With 15 against 15 I've no doubt in my mind that Wales would have won.'

I must remember to ask Derwyn, my agent, what he thinks about that last one. When Wales played South Africa in 1995, Derwyn was laid out by a peach of a haymaker. The man who threw that punch? Kobus Wiese.

Monday, 17 October. Turns out that I needn't worry about the reaction back home either. The front page of today's *Western Mail* carries no picture, just a message from the editor.

Is this how you feel?

Can't sleep.

Can't stop thinking about the game.

Can't stop imagining what a great week this would have been in Wales.

Can't stop mentally replaying the missed kicks in the hope that this time they'll clear the posts.

Can't stop wishing there had been a different referee.

Can't stop thinking he should have issued a yellow card, not a red one.

Can't stop questioning why he took such a short time to make such a big call.

Can't stop feeling his decision showed little empathy for the players, the occasion and the game.

Can't stop wanting to ask the ref 'Why?'

Can't stop feeling sad, proud and angry.

Can't watch any replays any more.

Can't stop being sure we'd have beaten France by a street without the sending off.

Can't stop concluding that the tournament has been devalued.

Can't stop believing we might have won the World Cup.

Can't stop believing in this truly magnificent team.

Warren Gatland's Wales – you've set the nation and the world alight. Thank you. Don't stop now.

Sunday, 23 October. Auckland. I'm here at Eden Park for the final. In a hospitality box rather than on the pitch, sadly.

I did my best for the boys in the week, providing opposition in training and being as positive as I could, but the disappointment had taken too much out of us. We gave it a go in the third place play-off, but Australia won 21–18. It wasn't a great game – the match is almost always an anti-climax – but it was at least a fair result, as the Wallabies were unquestionably the better team on the day.

I'm here with my folks, but for all of us it feels rather hollow. I can't remember much about the match other than the French making an arrowhead to face down the haka, Dusautoir tackling himself to a standstill, and New Zealand being nervous and very lucky to squeak home by a single point, the same margin by which France beat us last week.

I watch McCaw lift the trophy aloft amid the flashbulbs and the celebrations, and I'm happy for him. At least now his own countrymen might bracket him where his talent belongs. But I think of how close a pretty average French team ran the All Blacks, and I look at McCaw and his team-mates, and all I can think is this.

Could have been us.

Would have been us.

Should have been us.

Tuesday, 25 October. I stayed out for the IRB end of tournament dinner last night, more to ensure there was at least one Welsh representative there than anything else, as all the boys had gone home already. Now the time has come for my flight home, and I'm travelling alone.

I sit in the corner of the Emirates business lounge. The French lads are all there, since they're on the same flight as me. I keep my head down, and only go to the gate at the very last call. When I board the plane I hear a few of them sniggering, which I think's a little disrespectful, but I don't rise to it.

I count off the rows as I walk down the aisle until I reach mine. The sniggering's a bit louder now. There's only one seat left, and guess who's sitting right next to it with a cheesy grin all over his face?

Vincent Clerc. Who else?

I start laughing too. Emirates have got a good sense of humour, I'll give them that. I sit down and shake Clerc's hand. 'Maybe you could give me a massage on my back?' he says with his sexy French accent.

We chat all the way from Auckland to Brisbane. He's a good bloke, and we both know we've been part of something big, something that rugby fans will remember for a long time. There are no hard feelings on either side.

At Brisbane the French lads catch a different plane, and I'm bumped up to first class. It's 12 hours to Dubai. I close the doors of my compartment and don't leave for the entire flight, not even for a pee. I'm shattered.

Wednesday, 26 October. I do five and a half hours of interviews straight when I arrive back in Cardiff. In each one I stick to the line I've used so far, that I agree with Rolland's decision to send me off, but actually deep down I don't. I think it should have been yellow, as that's how most of the games were being officiated. Other incidents in that tournament which were worse than mine didn't lead to red cards. Yellow, I'd have had no problem with. The red seems too harsh.

But there's no point saying so in public. It won't change anything, and it'll just stir up the controversy again.

Monday, 31 October. Derwyn is round my house, and we have plenty to talk about: the media interest not just in the team but in me personally has gone through the roof. It's Halloween, though, and we can't get more than a moment's peace without the doorbell ringing.

Each time I get up, open the door and give some sweets to the trick-or-treaters, but increasingly I realise it's not just kids who are there but their parents too, taking pictures of me with their cameras or on their phones.

'This is really starting to hack me off,' I tell Derwyn after about the twentieth interruption.

The doorbell goes again.

'I'll get it,' Derwyn says.

Derwyn's 6 ft 10, with a bald head and a big bushy beard. He looks frightening at the best of times, let alone when he actually wants to be.

He opens the door and growls at the crowd. They leg it even quicker than the waiter in Auckland.

In his book *Calon: A Journey to the Heart of Welsh Rugby*, the playwright, poet and author Owen Sheers described me at that World Cup as 'the first onto the training pitch, the first to put on his recovery skins, to make his protein shake or to fill the ice bath. Under his captaincy "no sapping" became the ethos of the team. If you're hurting, tell the physios, but not your teammates. If you're tired, tell the conditioning coaches, but not the other players. If the English squad at the tournament were displaying the qualities of Prince Hal in *Henry IV Part I* – going out drinking, being careless with their reputations – then Sam and his team were more like the young king of *Henry IV Part II*: determined, ruthless and choosing to harness their youth for the fight, not the revels.'

You can't change the past. But if I had a time machine and only one opportunity to use it, this is the one I'd alter. We were so close, and yet we should have been even closer. Of course it would have been great for me to captain a side to the World Cup and join a pretty illustrious list of names – David Kirk, Nick Farr-Jones, François Pienaar, John Eales, Martin Johnson and John Smit. And of course it would have been great for the Welsh fans and public.

But most of all, it would have been great for rugby. It would have shaken things up a bit, for a tiny country to have won it. It would have shown that you don't always need to be one of the big nations to succeed. It would have broken the four-way monopoly on the trophy: only New Zealand, Australia, South Africa and England have ever won it. It would have given hope to every team, no matter how much of an underdog they might be – this could be your victory, this could be your time, today could be your day.

It could so nearly have been. It wasn't to be. But we gave it a damn good shot.

LEADERSHIP 3: PERFORMANCE

It's very easy as a captain to find your own performance levels slipping. You have so many more responsibilities than your team-mates, particularly off the field, and these can eat up your time and your focus. This applies across many sports, not just rugby. Tour de France leaders have to do hours of media after each day's stage when they'd rather be recovering; cricketers often find their averages declining quite sharply when they're captain.

Having to think about more than your own personal performance can be distracting, and at times can require two diametrically opposite mindsets – for me before a match, the distinction between my player headspace (ready to kill someone) and my captain headspace (talk to the ref and opposing captain, be nice to the terrified mascot, remember to ask them their name and what school they go to). And you're under much more scrutiny than your team-mates, so even the slightest loss of form is immediately noticed, seized upon and dissected.

As a leader, you need to maintain your own performance levels, not just for the team's sake – they can't afford to be carrying a passenger – but for your own too. If you're not pulling your weight in your own personal tasks, you'll begin to lose respect from the others, no matter how well you're performing your leadership role.

How do you go about doing this? By knowing when to be selfish. Sometimes the best way, maybe the only way, of being a selfless leader is to be selfish.

For example, you have to prioritise. When there are lots of competing demands on your time, assess each of them according to two criteria: importance and urgency. If something's important but doesn't need doing now, don't do it. If something needs doing now but isn't important, don't do it. If something's neither important nor urgent, definitely don't do it! Only if something's both important and urgent should you do it.

I tried to apply this to my own career. Let's take a day during my playing career in which my schedule had ten things listed:

- Weights session
- Skills session
- Mental affirmation session with Andy
- Physio session
- Senior players' meeting
- Referee meeting
- Sponsor photoshoot
- Charity appearance
- Press conference
- Social night out

Clearly, if I had to do every one of these things I'd be running from pillar to post all day, which would give me no time to rest – and knowing when to rest is as important as knowing when to work, as no one can drive themselves indefinitely without seeing a drop-off in their performance levels and decision-making.

So which ones to ditch? Or, conversely, which ones are essential?

Anything directly connected to the core task is essential. In this instance, the core task was personal performance on the pitch, and the first four of these ten commitments – weights, skills, mental affirmation and physio – are all directly connected to that. So they stay.

The next two, the meetings with senior players and referee, were also connected to events on the pitch, but less directly. Ideally, I'd like to be at both, but do I really need to be? If I have to choose one and ditch one, which should I choose? It would depend on the circumstances. If there was a pressing issue the senior players wanted to discuss, then I would go there and let Gats and the other coaches deal with the referee. If the senior players' meeting was a routine one and there was a specific issue I wanted to raise with the referee, then vice versa.

The final four are not directly connected to events on the pitch, but my responsibilities extend quite a long way off the pitch too. With sponsor photoshoots and charity appearances, there's a large contractual element: both of these things are written into the terms of player agreements, though of course you can do extra on both fronts. If neither was mandatory, I'd ask whether one or more of the other boys could do it, not least because I didn't want people just seeing me and a couple of other faces the whole time.

Particularly in the charity case, it would be important that it was a charity to which I felt personally attached and to which I could devote proper time. I could have spent each and every day doing charity work, but I never wanted to swan in and out of lots of different places. I wanted to give not just my profile but my time and effort too.

That leaves the press conference and the social night out. For the press conference, I'd ask if they really needed me or whether someone else could do it. If something to do with the captaincy was on the agenda, then of course it would be important for me to go; but if not, why not ask someone else? It wouldn't even have to be one of the senior boys. Ask one of the younger guys in the squad; it would be good for their confidence and give the press someone new to write about.

As for the social night out – well, I'm such an antisocial so-and-so that I'd almost certainly give it a miss anyway. Sometimes you need to go for team harmony, but if it's just a bog-standard night when some boys are going out and others aren't, I'd rather get some room service and rest.

So these ten events are now down to about six, which is much more manageable. But of course whittling them down involves having to say no. Some people find this easy, perhaps unnervingly so. But for others, myself included, saying no is much harder. You want to help, you want to be available, you don't want to let people down, and so the temptation is to say yes.

Andy helped me here too, even going so far as to give me a sheet of excuses! When someone would ask me to do something, I'd tell them I had to look at my diary, or check with my agent. That would buy me time to really consider what would be needed of me and whether I could justify doing it.

The flip side of stopping your personal performance from slipping is guarding yourself against any kind of complacency. Whether with Wales or the Lions, I never assumed I was going to be picked just because I was captain. This was another of the reasons I chose not to sit on selection committees. I liked going into team announcements and being on the edge like everyone else, not knowing whether I'd be picked or not.

For example, my birthday fell before the quarter-final against Ireland in 2011. I was sitting down at the dinner table with all the other players when in walked Huw Bennett with a huge cake, and all the boys started singing 'Happy Birthday'. It was a nice moment, but then when the cake was cut I didn't know whether to have a piece or not. A few days out from the match, when I was in great shape, a slice wouldn't have made any difference to me physically. But it would have made a difference to me *mentally*. Before every game I need to know in my own mind that I've done everything possible to prepare myself. Chocolate is my treat after a game, but not before. If I broke that rule, it would have been easier to break the next one, and the next, and suddenly those standards I'd always set myself would have been slipping. Not by much, but that's irrelevant. Either you set standards or you don't, and when you set them you have to abide by them.

My commitment to personal performance also manifested itself in a way some people found a little strange: that I'd never ask my opposite number if they wanted to swap shirts. For me, asking that question implied offering them a respect I didn't want to show. I didn't want McCaw, for example, to think that I'd been grateful for the opportunity to play against him (even though a man who played 148 Tests would hardly miss the odd shirt or two).

McCaw must have played an endless line of young punks who wanted to show him they were the real deal. But in my own eyes,

I *was* the real deal. I didn't need to be grateful to play against him or anyone else. I didn't want to be craven. I wanted him to think he was playing against an equal. It's not that I didn't think any of my opponents weren't good: of course they were. It was just that I wanted to be better.

That said, I always swapped shirts with someone if they asked. Without wanting to sound arrogant, the shirt of a Wales and Lions captain is a big deal for someone who plays for a lower-level team like Uruguay or Namibia, and who may not even be a full-time professional. I genuinely enjoyed playing those matches and meeting those guys, so it was a pleasure to swap shirts.

And I was pretty happy after one of the matches we played against Australia when Pocock came into our dressing-room and asked to swap, because of all the men I played against he was the one I admired most, not just as a player (he was consistently my most difficult opponent, and the only one I think who got the better of me over the course of all the matches we played) but also as a man (he's an outspoken activist on several issues, including gay rights and the environment).

His shirt, along with those of every player who's swapped, reminds me of the essential truth about performance. There are no armbands on those shirts, no indication whether or not the wearer was captain. There's just a number on the back, and that number signifies that the wearer was good enough to play for his country on that day. If that's not the case, then no leadership in the world can make up for it.

4

MILLENNIUM STADIUM

51.4782°N, 3.1826°W

**Saturday, 16 March 2013. Wales v England,
Six Nations decider**

*I'm ready to pile in as first man into the ruck when I see
something.*

They've got no one sweeping.

*I scoop the ball up and burst through the middle. The crowd
roar is like a tsunami at my back. I look right, then left. The
speed and suddenness of my burst has taken even my team-
mates by surprise. All I can see are white shirts: seven of them,
some muddied and dirty and others still pristine, scrambling
back behind me.*

Ten metres. Twenty. Run, Forrest. Run.

*Farrell's up ahead, waiting for me. He goes high. Too high. I
half-shrug him off and keep going a few more paces with him
clinging onto my neck until Tom Croft arrives to help him
bring me down.*

*Phillsy fires it out fast while England are still scrambling.
Justin with Cuthie outside him and Mike Brown trying to*

cover both of them. Justin drawing Brown, throwing the dummy and keeping on. Brad Barritt half-catching Justin, letting Brown make the tackle second time round, but Cuthie's still on Justin's shoulder and he takes the pass to go in untouched.

Still on my hands and knees 40 metres away, I punch the ground as hard as I can.

Game, set, match, championship.

Rach and I go out for a meal. I'm asked for three autographs even before the starter's arrived, and then when it does come and I've got a mouthful of food, some bloke just plonks himself down and puts his arm around me so his mate can take a photo. The autographs I don't mind, but the photo I do. No one looks their best while eating. Just ask Ed Miliband and his bacon sandwich.

It's a far cry from that moment in St David's 2 after my first home game two years ago – *only* two years ago – when Rach and I giggled at my being recognised by a solitary person. There aren't that many places in Cardiff where I won't be bothered now.

I buy a drum kit and thrash away on it for hours on end to let off some steam. Dad approves. He's got about 600 heavy metal albums, and always says drumming's the heartbeat of that kind of music. When I'm playing I imagine myself as some kind of rock god, but in reality I probably look like Animal from *The Muppet Show*.

Rach tries to get me reading, but I'm more interested in watching property shows on TV. I love real estate. Ryan and

Shane have got their own letting agency, and I pick their brains about the property market whenever we're in training camp. If this whole rugby thing doesn't work out, I'd like to pursue a career in that kind of field.

Sunday, 5 February 2012. First match of the Six Nations, in Dublin against an Ireland side still smarting from the World Cup quarter-final. It's another immensely physical, take-no-prisoners game. I get a dead leg in the first half, and at half-time the physios assess it and tell me I'm off.

A dead leg might not sound much – it's the kind of thing kids try to give each other in the school playground – but its more technically known as a thigh contusion, a crushing of the muscle against the bone which tears the fibres of that muscle and makes the leg hard to move.

Injury #6.

I watch the entire second half from the bench. With 15 minutes to go, Bradley Davies tip tackles Donnacha Ryan off the ball. It's much worse than the one for which I was sent off in the World Cup semi-final four months ago, and Bradley's very, very lucky that the card Wayne Barnes shows him is yellow rather than red.

By the time Bradley comes back on with five minutes to go, we're six points down, but George North scores in the corner to bring it back to within a point, and with less than a minute left we're awarded a penalty bang in front of the posts. Pence nails it, and we squeak home.

Saturday, 25 February. Having missed our win against Scotland through that injury, I'm raring to go against England at Twickenham. If we win this, we win the Triple Crown too, and of course keep our Grand Slam hopes alive.

Twenty-seven minutes gone, 3–3. England have a lineout and scorch upfield, moving it fast through the hands: Dylan Hartley on the run around, Dave Strettle off his wing into midfield, Brad Barritt running hard on the outside shoulder. It takes three men – Foxy, Phillsy and Pence – to bring Barritt down, and already they're looking to move it wide, so I haven't got time to go all the way around the ruck. I come into the defensive line from an offside position, turning to keep an eye on the play as I do so, and by the time Lee Dickson dive passes out to the England left I'm just about onside.

They're ten metres out with a man over and we're scrambling. I'm waving defenders over to my side but we haven't got enough. Faz (Owen Farrell) shuffles left and passes to Manu Tuilagi. I'm on Tuilagi's inside shoulder and outside me there's only Cuthie (Alex Cuthbert) drifting with two men on him, so I have to make this tackle, I simply have to.

He's a unit. Go low on him. Go high and he'll just bounce me off. Go low on him and don't let go. Close your eyes and dive at his ankles.

I'm side-on to Tuilagi as he hammers towards the line. Full stretch as I dive at him, head first and willing to break my nose if that's what it takes. I wrap my arms round his ankles and he hits the ground. *Keep holding on. Don't let him get up.* He tries to bounce himself forward but I'm still there, and now we've got men in the ruck and I'm leaping up to take up the guard position on the blindside and they're having to work it back the other way towards the open spaces.

At the time, I don't think anything of that tackle. I know it's technically a good one and saved a try, but it's also the kind of tackle I practise in training several times a week and one I'd always back myself to make.

It's only after the match, which we win 19–12 to secure the Triple Crown, that I find the world and his wife wanting to congratulate me on it.

I sprain my medial knee ligament during that game and have to sit out our victory against Italy at the Millennium a fortnight later.

Injury #7.

Sunday, 17 March. Cardiff, and we're four wins from four matches. This one's for the Grand Slam, and who else can our opponents be but France? Not a single player on either side will forget what happened the last time we met. Winning today won't erase the pain of that defeat, but losing is also unthinkable. Winning four games out of five is a hell of an achievement in any Six Nations, but if the one you lose is the very last one when you're going for a Slam … it must take a long time to get over the hurt, put it that way.

Five things will secure us the win and the Slam, Shane says. Attack their scrum, change the points of our attack, and keep the tempo high, nullify their back row, and stick to our game plan.

The first half is frantic and scrappy. We come in at the break 10–3 up, but for me the game and the tournament are both over. I've damaged a nerve in my right shoulder, and my arm on that side is more or less useless. There's no way I can carry on.

What is it about the French? Three times I've played them now, and not once have I finished the match. The knee injury in the Stade de France last year, the red card at Eden Park and now this.

We hang on to beat them 16–9 and win the Slam. Lyds is voted player of the tournament, which is richly deserved, and I'm absolutely chuffed for my great mate. But when I lift the trophy with my left arm – my right arm is hanging down immobile by my side – I don't really feel I deserve to be the one holding it. Of the five matches in this year's tournament, I've only effectively played two whole ones: the first half against Ireland, the match against England and the first half against France. Forty per cent of the total time I could have played.

Three months out, the doctors say. Injury #8.

Friday, 25 May. I carry the Olympic torch past the Millennium Stadium as part of the Cardiff section of the relay. The crowds are cheering and clapping, and their reaction makes me certain that the Games will be a huge success when they start in a couple of months' time, despite all the grumbling about the cost, the disruption and how many things will go wrong.

Saturday, 26 May. The *Western Mail* carries a big picture of me with the Olympic torch. One for the scrapbook, I guess, apart from the small matter of the headline directly below the photograph.

PAEDOPHILE JAILED AFTER 12 YEARS ON THE LOOSE.

Saturday, 23 June. Sydney. Wales summer tour of Australia, Third Test. Less than half an hour gone, and I know my game is over. I come off to be replaced by Justin Tipuric, a man who many people think should have started the match in my place.

It's been a pretty miserable tour all told. We lost the first Test in Brisbane 27–19, and the second Test last week in Melbourne by two points right at the end, with Mike Harris kicking an injury-time penalty when we thought that for once we'd managed to hold on in a tight game against Australia. That was the series gone, and in an hour or so's time the Wallabies will sneak another narrow win – by even less this time, a single point – to close out the whitewash.

If it's been miserable for the team, it's been just as miserable for me. I've only just come back from the injury I sustained against France, and I always need a few games to get back into form, but I haven't had that luxury here.

And if there's one guy you don't want to be playing against when you're not on top of your game, it's Pocock. He's done a number on me in all three Tests, properly outplaying me. At my best, I'm a match for him; but I'm not, far from it.

Justin, on the other hand, is very much at his best, or very near to it. That's why there's such a groundswell of support for him to take my place. It's a debate that won't really go away for the rest of my career. It's like the Beatles and the Stones, or Blur and Oasis; people tend to support one or other of us, whether it's for Wales or the Lions.

Even though we play in the same position, we're very different types of player. Justin plays more as a link man between forwards and backs. His hands and feet are quick enough for him to play 13 at international level, his levels of aerobic fitness are ludicrous – he and Bradley are the two best natural athletes I've ever played with – and his form for the Ospreys week in, week out is consistently good.

I'm stronger over the ball in the jackal and when hitting people in the tackle, and the ultra-physical way I play means I can't put in big matches for the Blues on a regular basis. The one area where we're both equally good is as lineout jumpers – indeed, in one Six Nations the two of us will end up with more lineout takes than anybody else, including our own second rows.

Certainly, Justin's strengths are more visible to the casual fan. He does more of his work in the open, whereas I do more of mine on the floor in a pile of bodies. People see him pop up in a move to provide the extra man and make space for the men outside him; they don't so often see the way I slow a ball down for just long enough to allow our defensive line to regroup. They don't see the tries that my breakdown work has prevented four or five phases earlier, because I've helped ensure those tries aren't scored in the first place.

But whether you're Team Warburton or Team Tipuric, I can't deny that right now Justin's in better form than I am. I've always relished challenges like this – nothing makes me raise my game like knowing that my position's under threat – but for once I'm beginning to doubt myself. The injuries have taken a lot out of me, as has the relentless physical grind: I've played 15 Test matches in the past year alone.

It's a constant drip, drip, drip: the erosion of everything good. Perhaps it's not that surprising. The margins are so slim at this level that no one can remain on top form indefinitely. McCaw puts it well when he says that we 'live in that split second of time and space at the breakdown, a collision zone where 100-plus kilogram bodies are hurtling from diverse points of the compass towards a small ovoid focus. Success or failure can be measured in microseconds. Openside flankers live or die in those slivers of time.'

But it's still frustrating, and it still eats away at me. Nine months ago, I could do no wrong. Now it seems I can't do much right.

I go away with Rach on holiday to west Wales. For these few weeks, between the end of one season and the start of the next, I'm emphatically not Sam Warburton, Wales captain and rugby player. I'm Sam Kennedy-Warburton, normal bloke.

We go for a walk in one of our favourite beauty spots. I go down on one knee and ask Rach to marry me. She starts crying. I have a moment of panic – I've got no Plan B if she says no – but through the tears she nods and says yes.

Amazingly, I manage to get through the whole thing without throwing up.

Saturday, 13 October. I dislocate the middle finger on my left hand six minutes into the Blues' match against Sale. The doctors in A&E pop it back in for me.

Injury #9.

Friday, 26 October. On the tarmac at Cardiff Airport, waiting to fly to Dublin where we'll play Leinster in the Pro12 tomorrow.

I'm looking out of the window at the marshal with his paddles, signalling the plane forwards. *If that bloke offered me a job swap, right now I'd bite his hand off. Why can't I have a job like that? Why can't I have a job with no outside stress, no pressure from others? Why do I put myself through this? If we lose again, I'm going to get slagged off again, and my parents and Rach will worry themselves sick about me again.*

Saturday, 27 October. We don't lose. Rather, we don't *just* lose. We get hammered. At half-time Leinster are leading 40–3, and though we make a slightly better fist of it in the second half, we're playing for pride and pride alone. The final score is 59–22. They put nine tries past us. Our performance is abject: there's no other word for it (at least not one you can use in polite company).

'That's the most embarrassing game I've ever played in,' I tell Jamie afterwards.

He nods in agreement. 'It was men against boys.'

·I don't see the aircraft marshal when we land back at Cardiff. Just as well. I'd probably grab the paddles off him and never let them go.

Time to stop the rot. We need to start winning again. We've got four autumn internationals at the Millennium on consecutive Saturdays – Argentina, Samoa, New Zealand and Australia – and we need to win at least the first two.

Saturday, 10 November. We're looking ponderous and tired, a far cry from the team that just a year ago was winning hearts across the rugby world at the World Cup. The last time I played for Wales in this stadium was against France in March, when the crowd had roared us to a Grand Slam. Now that same crowd turns on us, booing as we go down to Argentina 26–12.

In the Millennium more than any other stadium, crowd and players are two sides of the same coin. When we're playing well, that energises the crowd, which in turn makes us play even better; but when we're playing badly, the crowd goes flat and truculent, which further saps the energy from our play.

Saturday, 17 November. The Samoa match is a war zone, as it often is against them. Hibbs (Richard Hibbard) and Dan Biggar are taken off injured in the first half; Ian Evans doesn't come out after half-time. With 15 minutes remaining we're ahead by a point, but they score a penalty and a try to run out 26–19 winners. More boos from the stands.

Saturday, 24 November. I've always prided myself on raising my game against the big boys, and they don't come any bigger than the All Blacks. We haven't beaten New Zealand since 1953, and that grim statistic never looks like being altered when we play them this time. They blow us away. They're 23–0 up at half-time, and though we share the second half 10–10, the damage has long been done.

I play much better than before, which is something. With ten minutes to go, I'm walking towards a lineout when I hear the crowd cheering for me. It brings tears to my eyes, it really does. Ten minutes left and I'm crying on the pitch with happiness that I've had a good game and some of the pressure will stop.

Saturday, 1 December. Now we have to beat the Wallabies, not just to salvage something from this campaign but also to purge the memory of their two last-ditch victories against us in the summer.

I'm fired up for this one, and it shows. Michael Hooper pins me to the floor by my jersey and won't let me go, even though the ball's nowhere near us. After that he's constantly chirping away, trying to get under my skin.

Suddenly, at another ruck, I've had enough. You know when people talk about seeing red? I really do – it's like the whole world's taken on the tinge of blood for a moment. I press my forehead against his and start throttling him as hard as I can. 'Touch me again and I'll cut your throat,' I hiss. Then I pick him up, throw him on his back and jog off to catch up with play. At the next scrum, I notice that I'm still shaking with aggression.

With one minute to go, we're 12–9 up. Surely we can't lose it from here, a third last-gasp defeat in a row? Sure we can. Kurtley Beale scoots in at the corner with 30 seconds to go, and Australia win 14–12.

'That's the worst defeat I've ever been involved with,' I tell the press. 'To be in control really for the majority of the second half, and in the last play of the game we slip up. It's really hard to take.'

It's also left us with another problem, the magnitude of which becomes apparent two days later.

Monday, 3 December. I'm at the Tate Modern gallery in London, along with pretty much every member of world rugby's great and good. It's the draw for the 2015 World Cup. Almost three years out from the tournament seems an awfully long time to be doing this, but the logic is that it allows the organisers to make provisions for the visiting fans and official travel firms to block-book hotels.

The downside, of course, is that an awful lot can happen on and off the pitch in three years, which can play havoc with the seeding. A team flying high right now may be on the skids by the time the tournament comes round, and vice versa. Three years is a long time to maintain your form. So the logic, as so often seems to be the case, suits the administrators more than the players.

Our seven defeats in a row – the three summer Tests and the four autumn internationals – mean that, as of the new IRB rankings published this morning, we're no longer in the top eight. Since the World Cup seedings are done in bands of four, this is a big deal.

We're now in Band 3, along with Italy, Tonga and Scotland. Each pool at the tournament will have five teams, one from each band, which means we'll have in our group one of the Band 2 countries (England, Ireland, Argentina and Samoa) and one of the Band 1 countries (New Zealand, Australia, South Africa and France).

They do the draw in reverse order. The countries in Bands 4 and 5 have yet to be determined; they're still going through their qualification games, and with respect they'll all be the kind of minnow teams who we'd back ourselves to beat every day of the week and twice on Sunday.

We're the first name out of Band 3. Into Pool A we go.

Now the Band 2 countries are being drawn. First out of the pot, and coming into Pool A with us, is ... England.

There's a ripple around the room, something between a communal gasp and a collective whistling. England v Wales in a pool match. Talk about spicy. The cameras focus on England coach Stuart Lancaster and his captain Chris Robshaw. They're both smiling, though quite how sincerely I can't really tell.

From Band 1 we get Australia. This is now the Group of Death; not just the hardest group of this World Cup but of any World Cup in history. Three into two doesn't go. Even at this distance, I'm absolutely determined we won't be the ones to miss out.

Saturday, 2 February 2013. The new year starts as the old one left off – terribly.

The Irish come to Cardiff for the Six Nations opener. For the first half at least, they pulverise us. Simon Zebo scores their first try and then helps set up the second with a breathtaking piece of skill: when Jamie Heaslip's pass goes low behind him, Zebo backheels it into his own hands without breaking stride. It's the kind of thing most players couldn't do in a hundred goes on a training pitch, let alone first time in a match.

The Irish are 23–3 up at half-time and extend that to 30–3 within two minutes of the restart. We're looking down the barrel of a fifth straight defeat at the Millennium and an eighth in all. Any hope of a second consecutive Grand Slam has also gone. With all that, you might think we'd crumble even further.

In fact, quite the opposite happens. It's as if we're liberated, as if everyone simultaneously goes, 'Ah, let's just play some

rugby.' And that's just what we do. We go back to basics, playing the percentages rather than trying to make every touch a
Hollywood one. We know we're better than this. Cuthie, Pence
and Craig Mitchell all score tries to bring us back to within
eight points, but Ireland hang on and we run out of time.
'Pride's a horrible beast,' Hibbs says, 'and a lot changes when
your pride's on the line.'

When you lose a match, you like to talk about taking positives from the defeat. Half the time that's just stuff you say for
the TV, but on this occasion it's true. The shift in momentum
during that second half is something that stays with us. Now
we've got three away games on the trot to the 'blue teams' –
France, Italy and Scotland. Tough asks, all of them, and we're
no longer defending a Grand Slam; in other words, we're back
under pressure, we're back with the underdogs, the place where
we play our best rugby.

When the BBC's Sonja McLaughlan tells me during the post-
match interview that no one's won the Six Nations after losing
their first match for 20 years – back when it was still the Five
Nations – my first thought is, *Well, records are there to be
broken*. The next day, Mike Averis writes some prophetic
words in the *Observer*: 'If Wales stop giving themselves ridiculous handicaps, they could still be in with a shout when the Six
Nations ends next month.'

For me personally, the match is doubly frustrating. First, I
don't get a single turnover, which is both rare and disappoint-
ing – I usually target three or four each game. Every time I get
over the ball in a ruck, the Irish double-team me and clean me
out. Every single time. Just as our back row did a number on
theirs at the World Cup 18 months earlier, now they return the

favour. They're definitely the alpha males today, and that hurts. But at least I'm still getting in those positions to compete for the ball. I'd be even more worried if I hadn't been making it to the rucks in the first place.

Second, I get a stinger injury. You know that feeling when you bite into ice-cream and the cold goes searing through your teeth? Imagine that, but from just below your ear all the way down your left shoulder and arm to the end of your fingers. Now imagine that lasting not just a couple of seconds but a couple of minutes. It feels like my arm's come out of my socket, and I can't move that arm or sense anything I'm touching with it. The reason it's my left arm is that I tend to lead with my right shoulder when I'm making big hits, which in turn makes my neck flex to the left, which in turn jams the vertebrae on that side and pinches the nerves there.

Injury #10.

I miss the next game, the win in Paris, and come off the bench for the last 12 minutes as we beat Italy in Rome. That we've done better without me than with me hasn't escaped people's notice, and once more the calls for me to be dropped start up again – not that they ever really went away, in some quarters at least. I try not to read most of the stuff, but that's harder than it seems; people send me links, or texts asking, 'Have you read what so-and-so's been saying?', and then curiosity gets the better of me and before I know it I'm spending hours online trawling through all the criticism.

And because often I can't see who's slagging me off – it's just anonymous people hiding behind usernames – I give some of the stuff more credence than I should. If a fat, pissed bloke came up to me outside a pub and said, 'Warburton, you're shit,' I'd just laugh, because I'd think, *You don't know the first thing about life as a professional rugby player, mate*. But if that same fat, pissed bloke is saying it online, and it happens to chime with some negative thoughts I'm feeling, then rather than laugh it off I find that those criticisms can actually reinforce my negative thoughts and make them worse.

As that professional rugby player – and this goes for pros in all sports – you live and die by your results. In most workplaces, being a few per cent off your best won't make much, if any, difference to your performance. But in professional sport those few percentage points can be the difference between being in the team or not, between having a contract or not, between having sponsor endorsements or not. That in turn means that your professional and your personal identities begin to merge. As long as you're doing well you're a good bloke, but as soon as you start to tail off you're a shit bloke. You can't rationalise it enough to separate one from the other.

And the logical endpoint of that is where I ended up while looking out of the window at Cardiff Airport, or marching into my in-laws' house to pick up the dog once, or in a Wellington hotel at two in the morning, or in the middle of a game, or on any of the other half-dozen occasions I've 'retired' in my career. You just want out, because you're tired of a life that seems so pressured and unreal.

I watch my local rugby club Rhiwbina play. No GPS chip in a little pouch on their shirts between the shoulder blades, no six-camera set-up capturing everything they do, no heart-rate monitoring, no analysis, no debrief other than piss-taking in the pub. It's so tempting. All of that is so, so tempting. I'd lose the sponsored car, but so what? I could drive an eight-year-old Ford, work nine to five and live for the weekend.

Snap out of it. Snap out of it now.

I've worked too hard to get to where I am just to give it all up. Winners never quit and quitters never win. Anyway, every-one's career has ups and downs. My time will come again, I'm sure of it. I *have* to be sure of it. I just don't know *when* it will come again.

Rob Howley comes to me before the Scotland match and says two things: that I'm starting at 7, and that Ryan Jones is going to be captain instead.

'Are you disappointed?' he asks.

I almost laugh. 'Disappointed? I'm delighted. To be honest, mate, I was going to have a word with you anyway. I need to get back to my old self as a player and a person. I want to be in the changing-room before a game and just listen to my crazy music for an hour, not say a word, and then go out and smash the opposition. That's how I approach my game best. I don't want to worry about press conferences or coin tosses or which way we should play or what I'm going to say to the players. I don't want any of that stuff. I just want to concentrate on myself and play as well as I can, because that's what'll be best for the team.'

There's another thing, of course. The reason Rob's in charge for this season is that Gats is head coach of the Lions tour to Australia this summer, and every Home Nations player wants to be on that plane with him.

No one mentions it out loud. It's almost a taboo: don't put a hex on it. There's a day when Cuthie writes his name on the massage sheet, to book himself a massage. Someone, just messing about, writes 'Lions 14' next to it. Cuthie comes back in, sees this, says, 'No chance' straight away and scribbles it out.

No one wants to say it, then, but everyone's thinking it. Everyone wants to play as well as they can, not just for their team but for their own chances of being picked for the Lions.

If the tour had been two years ago, I'd have been a shoo-in. Now, I'm not so sure. Yes, I played well against Australia and New Zealand in the autumn, but the Ireland game last month did me no favours, and nor did sitting out the best part of the two matches since then. I've got two opportunities left to shine. The Scotland and England matches aren't just vital for Wales's chances of winning the championship; they're vital for my chances of making the Lions trip.

And the Lions, even more than Wales, is what I've always dreamed about.

Derwyn, for one, knows this full well. At the height of the criticism of me, when every bloke with a smartphone and an internet connection is weighing in, he sends me a picture of a lion staring down the camera with blood dripping from its mouth.

'Lions don't worry about the opinions of sheep,' says the caption.

Thursday, 7 March. I'm doing a session with Andy.

'What's your target for the Scotland match?'

'To be man of the match.'

'That's fine. But what if, even though you have a man-of-the-match performance, the commentary people selecting it don't see it that way?'

'Then I'm going to have that good a game that they can't ignore me.'

Saturday, 9 March. It's cold, grey and windy at Murrayfield; practically tropical by local standards, in other words.

The match is a dogfight, scrappy and disjointed from the start. We go in at half-time 13–12 up. I'm playing well enough, making my tackles and hitting rucks. I'm solid without being outstanding, but I need more. I need to make an impact. A proper impact, the kind of impact the old Sam Warburton – the *real* Sam Warburton – would make.

The real Sam Warburton. Find him, and everything else will fall into place.

I'm looking down the barrel here. I'm not thinking about this match, and I'm certainly not thinking about the Lions. I'm thinking about me. Me, and me alone. The coaches are bustling around, talking. I don't hear what they're saying. I know what I need to do.

I clamp my headphones on: Anthrax, as loud and angry as I can make them.

Refuse to be denied.

Refuse to compromise.

The guitar, the drums, the singer screaming. Slamming in with the first drumbeat, twatting the nearest bloke. You may as well give up now, mate. No way you're beating me. No way.

Drum, slam. Drum, slam. Drum, slam.

Refuse to be denied.

Refuse to be denied.

Refuse to be denied.

I come out for the second half like a snarling dog.

Two minutes after the restart. Scotland coming from deep, counter-attacking at pace. Duncan Weir feeds Stuart Hogg. I line Hogg up, stand him up, drive him back, take him to the floor and grab the ball as I jackal. Four Scottish players come piling in to help, but I'm still there, strong over the ball, almost smiling as the hits come in. Bang, bang, bang, bang. *Still here, lads. Still here.*

Ref Craig Joubert whistles. Penalty against Hogg for holding on. 'That's Warburton at his best,' Jiffy (Jonathan Davies) says on the commentary. 'Great hit, stays on his feet.' Alun Wyn, Ianto (Ian Evans), Phillsy, Ryan, Hibbs – they all tap me on the head in congratulations as I get up.

I'm back.

Suddenly, I feel as if I can do anything. I'm a different player: quicker to the breakdown, stronger over the ball, harder in the tackle. Adrenaline coursing through me. I'm everywhere now, winning turnovers and penalties as though I'm on a mission – which, of course, I am. With 90 seconds to go and Scotland camped on our line as we defend a 10-point lead, I win another penalty jackalling on Kelly Brown. 'Sam Warburton has been absolutely immense in this game,' Jiffy says as he awards me man of the match, just as I'd told Andy I wanted to be.

After the match, I walk round the stadium with my man-of-the-match medal on. It feels like a talisman, an amulet; not just a reminder of the player I really am, but a huge middle finger to all the doubters. I walk round with it on until I find Mum and Dad in the stands, and I give it to them. They've suffered so much, not just from seeing all the negativity aimed at me but also from seeing my reaction to it. This medal is for them.

I think back to how low I've been feeling, and how that second half against Scotland has chased away the despair. The darkest hour is just before the dawn.

Tuesday, 12 March. It's Shaun's Tuesday afternoon drill to check that we're mentally primed, making us run into guys holding tackle pads for a minute at full chat. They're standing on four corners of a grid, and there's no hiding place. Smash them, smash them again, smash them again. 'I want to see you twat people,' Shaun shouts. 'I want to see that you're up for it.'

England, this Saturday, going for the Grand Slam, in our backyard. Oh, we're up for it. We're up for it all right.

Thursday, 14 March. Gethin does the press conference, as he's captain for this game. Ryan's injured, and when Rob asked me if I'd take the role again I said no. Concentrating on myself worked against Scotland. I want it to work against England too.

Ryan being out means that I'll take his position at 6 and Justin will play 7. After all the debate about which one of us is better, now we get to go in tandem. We're both in form. Let's take it to England. Let's destroy them at the breakdown.

All week it's been building, and still it builds. Security at the training ground to prevent our sessions from being watched. Fans hanging around the team hotel night and day, hoping for a glimpse of us, maybe an autograph or a selfie. We feed off the energy, but we have to be careful not to peak too soon. For a match like this, it's easy to get so worked up in advance that by the time match day comes round you're tailing off down the other side of your mental peak. The match is when it is. Don't play it too early.

The team room one level below ground is our sanctuary. Only players and management are allowed in here. This is where we have team meetings, and meals, and massages. This is where the daily schedules are posted, so everyone knows where they're supposed to be at any given time. This is where we wall ourselves off from the world outside, but somehow the excitement still percolates through the walls as if by osmosis. The press, the fans, the public; this game is special, and they all know it as well as we do.

Saturday, 16 March. Six days in the week, I give all the time I can to the fans. The seventh day, today, is mine. Today, I don't go through the foyer to and from the team room. Today, I use the rear car park and the underground tunnel the cleaners take. I have my routine, and it's timed down to the minute. Breakfast, nap, lunch, shower, all timed.

This is the worst time, the period between waking up and getting to the stadium. Today's an afternoon game, which is at least better than a night game. Night games are the worst, as you have the whole day to kill. If it were up to me I'd wake up, bolt down a couple of protein shakes, go out and play first thing, and have it all done and dusted by midday.

These hours are where the nerves really worm their way down into me. I know what I'll need to put my body through, and it scares me. I make half-bargains in my head. Give me food poisoning so I can't play. Let the bus crash – not badly, obviously – so I can't play. Let me turn my ankle on the stairs so I can't play. Let the game be snowed off, or the pitch waterlogged, or something like that. Unlikely beneath the Millennium's roof, I grant you.

Three hours until kick-off. We eat the pre-match meal in silence. Normally, team meals are loud and raucous, full of banter and blokes chopsing off good-naturedly at each other. Not today. Today the only sounds are the clanking of cutlery, the high ping of metal on china.

Two hours until kick-off. Our final team meeting. Some of the boys are there early, eyes half-closed as they listen to music in their headphones. Others filter in a few minutes ahead of time. Jamie and Toby come in last with 30 seconds to go, just like they always do. No one is ever late.

Rob slides his chair back and stands up.

'We're too big, too physical and too good for them. They're not as fit as you are, they're not as strong, they're not as skilful. They haven't got the experience you have, they haven't got the mental toughness you have. You're working-class lads from normal families, from the valleys. This is your turf. Let's go.'

On the team bus. 'TEAM WALES' and the dragon plastered across the sides, loud and proud of who we are. All the boys with their headphones on. Twelve miles from here to the stadium. Police outriders performing their strangely beautiful ballet, leapfrogging each other to hold traffic in the side roads and let us pass. Their lights reflect along the aisle down the middle of the bus: red and blue, red and blue, red and blue.

The drivers of the cars we pass honk their horns and pump their fists as we pass. On the outskirts of Cardiff the traffic's thin, but gradually both roads and pavements begin to fill as we approach the stadium. There are air horns now, and flags, and daffodil hats and replica shirts and face paint, and one by one we take our headphones off so we can watch and hear the crowds, because this is firing us up more than any music ever could.

T-shirts on sale. **ENGLAND: GRAND SLAM CHAMPIONS 2013.** The muscles in my jaw clench so hard you could crack walnuts with them. You know where you can stick your T-shirt, don't you, mate?

We reach the bottom of Westgate Street. It's pedestrianised from here on in, to the stadium a few hundred metres away. We're the only vehicle allowed on here. Two police horses walk slowly ahead of us through crowds 15 or 20 deep. It's a sea of red, thousands of people all packed into this one street, cheering and waving and clapping.

It wasn't like this for the match against Ireland last month, or for the autumn internationals, or even for the Grand Slam match against France last year. This is something else entirely, and I know without even needing to ask that not a single one of the squad will ever have experienced anything remotely like it before.

This is one of the best things about the Millennium: that it's right in the middle of Cardiff. Every other Six Nations stadium – Twickenham, Murrayfield, the Aviva, the Stade de France, the Stadio Olimpico – is away from the city centre. You can be in London, or Edinburgh, or Dublin, or Paris, or Rome on match day and not know the game's going on.

In Cardiff, you *know*. Everybody knows. And so it's not just that the stadium becomes the city, but also that the city becomes the country. Trains with extra carriages bolted on have been bringing people in from Abergavenny and Aberystwyth, from Bangor and Bridgend, from Cardigan and Colwyn Bay, and from a hundred other places too. Many of these people don't even have tickets for the match; they just want to be here, in the capital, when it's happening, to watch it on giant screens or in pubs, to feed off and contribute to this insane electricity pulsing through the city's streets.

These are the people cheering us on. These are the people we're playing for.

We turn right and follow the road down into the bowels of the stadium. Darkness, and the sounds of the crowd fading behind us. We get off the bus and head for the stairs that will take us up to the changing-room, and as we do we hear something so quintessentially Welsh they should bottle it and sell it at Cardiff Airport: a male voice choir, here just for us, singing 'Calon Lân'.

Nid wy'n gofyn bywyd moethus,
Aur y byd na'i berlau mân;
Gofyn wyf am galon hapus,
Calon onest, calon lân.

I don't ask for a luxurious life,
the world's gold or its fine pearls;
I ask for a happy heart,
an honest heart, a pure heart.

Calon lân yn llawn daioni,
Tecach yw na'r lili dlos;
Dim ond calon lân all ganu
Canu'r dydd a chanu'r nos.

A pure heart full of goodness
Is fairer than the pretty lily;
None but a pure heart can sing,
Sing in the day and sing in the night.

Their voices carry us all the way to the changing-room. On one wall, in three-foot-high red letters, is written 'RESPECT THE JERSEY'. On the opposite wall, in the same lettering, is 'DAL DY DIR'. 'Hold your ground'.

We take up the places marked out by our numbers. Inside the collar of the shirts hanging from the pegs is a single word. *Braint*. Privilege.

And right in the middle of the room – without telling any of us, Rob's asked for it to be put here, knowing the effect it will have on us – is the Six Nations trophy, sparkling clean and gleaming like the most precious of metals.

Our trophy.

Our trophy, which we won last year. Our trophy, which we're still defending, even though the possibility of a second Grand Slam went out of the window almost before it had started.

We know the maths. England have four wins, we have three. They also have a superior points difference. Beating them will deny them the Grand Slam, but to win the championship a simple victory won't be enough. To win the championship, we have to beat them by eight points.

Joe Lydon, the WRU's head of rugby, told us what his England Under-18s coach had once said. 'When you play Wales, remember that they're not defending their tryline. They're defending their border.'

Every single one of us has that thought right now, looking at the trophy.

No way. No way is that trophy going back across the Severn Bridge tonight.

Grim faces. Growls, shouts, murmurs. Studs clattering on the floor. The smell of liniment and fear. Tape being ripped and wound and ripped again. Hugs and backslaps. Energy gels, sickly sweet. Blokes spewing in the toilets.

An official's voice at the door. Two minutes. Two minutes.

Another voice. England are already in the tunnel. They're waiting for you. They don't want to go out alone.

Let them wait. We go when the ref tells us to, not a moment before.

Wales out, please. Wales out.

Single file in the corridor, looking at the back of the man in front of you. Something very literal in that: knowing that you've got his back just as the guy behind you has got yours.

Thick double doors between you and the playing arena. The crowd noise a distant thunder, rumbling and muffled, as though we're underwater. They can see us on the screen. They know we're coming.

Ten seconds, the TV guy says. Ten seconds.

The doors open. The noise is like a chemical blast, breaking down and over us. Red lights and dry ice in our faces. We can't

144

see further than the end of our arms, but we can hear everything, and we can feel it too. Pressure waves of sound, bouncing and reverberating and sloshing like water in a bath.

Then the dry ice clears, and suddenly the entire far side of the stadium comes into view: three tiers climbing to the heavens, wall upon wall of red. Our people.

Lining up for the anthems. The players' wives and girlfriends have two rows earmarked for them on halfway, always in the same place. Each time I play here, I look for Rach during the anthems, and each time she smiles at me. Our little routine: *I'm here for you, go on, play your heart out.*

The English anthem is first. 'God Save the Queen', and God it's loud. I've never heard it sung so loud. How the hell did so many English fans get in here? The place must be full of them. How's our anthem ever going to compete with that? This is going to be embarrassing. Outsung by England before the match has even started – for any proud Welshman that's humiliation right there.

Then 'Hen Wlad Fy Nhadau' starts up.

Wow.

Just wow.

No matter how loud the English had sung, that was nothing compared with this. Nothing. It sounds like the whole country's singing, not just the whole stadium. It raises not only the hairs on the back of my neck but all the way down my spine too. It's so loud that for a moment I wonder if the stadium can contain it, whether the walls will crumble like those of Jericho did at the sound of Joshua's trumpets. I don't sing the anthem – I never sing it – but inside I'm there with every word, lifted somewhere up into the gods up near the roof.

I glance across at the English boys. They're not that much younger than we are, but they're a lot less experienced: their starting XV has fewer than half the caps ours does. For quite a few of them, this is their first time playing in Cardiff. Hell of a game to choose to break your duck.

You poor bastards. You don't know what's about to hit you. You don't have a clue. And you don't have a prayer.

Owen Farrell kicks off for England. Phillsy catches it, it comes back to Dan Biggar who kicks to halfway, and when Farrell tries a grubber to the corner he overhits it and Pence touches down behind the line for a 22.

Normally, the crowd noise from the kick-off subsides by the first break in the play, if not before. Not today. The noise just keeps going and going, an almost unbroken wall of sound, and so does the game. It's fast and furious, and there's no let-up, not even for a moment, no chance of hearing the lineout calls, so we use body language. Alun Wyn's the caller, and we watch where he puts his hands or feet as we line up. Those are our cues, drilled into us all week.

I'm jumping in this lineout. Point your toes down, stiffen your glutes and tense your arse, that's Alun Wyn's advice; it stiffens your core and keeps you like a pencil. The lifters throwing me so high that they let me go and I'm still travelling upwards, 12 feet up and climbing, half as high again as a fullback jumping for a bomb, watching the ball all the way.

Hit the rucks as hard as I can. Split-second decisions as I arrive: where's the ball, where are the opposition, where's the next threat coming from? If there's someone there I've got to melt him, unload on him, punish him. Front rows might have to wait 10 or 15 minutes until the first scrum, but there are rucks all the time. Rucks are back-row manna. Hit each one as though it's the last one I'll ever hit.

Pence knocks over a penalty, and then another, to make it 6–0. Ianto tackles Barritt, and I'm the first man into the ruck, trying to steal the ball. Referee Steve Walsh whistles: penalty against me. I ask why. 'Straight on the ball, not past it,' he says. I ask why again, partly because it's so hard to hear him above the crowd. 'You were past the ball with your hands on the ground and went back onto the ball. You've got to go straight onto it.'

Walsh isn't a referee who likes to give explanations, let alone to someone who's not even the captain that day. Though obviously I don't know this at the time, up in the stands Gats makes a note – a note that will have big repercussions in a month or so's time.

Farrell nails the kick: 6–3.

The English front row pops up in a scrum, and Pence does the rest: 9–3.

Big hits coming in all over the park. Hibbs puts one in on Joe Marler that wouldn't be out of place in a wildlife documentary. George escapes down the wing and for a moment looks to be in, but Mike Brown throws himself headlong in desperation and makes the tap tackle. England coming at us, but their passing's too slow and we're keeping our shape and numbers well. Dan tries a drop goal from 30 metres out, but it fades just wide of the posts.

Half-time. Still 9–3. Anyone's game. And anyone's championship, too. As things stand we'll win the match but England will win the title.

Both sides pick up where they left off. Slowly, surely, we're beginning to put the squeeze on them, especially in the set piece. Tom Youngs is chirping as we set ourselves. Walsh is having none of it. 'Be quiet and scrum,' he says.

Little cracks in the England psyche. We have to crowbar them wide open. *We're fitter than they are, and we've had a day's more recovery than they have. Keep them moving. Keep them tackling. Keep the ball in play. We might be breathing through our arses, but they'll be worse. No matter how much we're feeling the pace, they'll be feeling it more.*

Our pressure, again and again. Jamie has a go, then Ianto, then Hibbs, then Jamie again. Walsh plays the advantage before taking us back for the penalty. Pence, cool as you like, nails it, 12–3, and for the first time we're virtual champions: that's a point more than we need.

It's not nearly enough for what we want, though. We want more, and so do the crowd. They can sense the English dam beginning to crack. Slim margins, but now we're doing the basics just that little bit better than they are, and in the end that's going to tell. It reminds me of Ireland in the 2011 quarter-final. There's not much in it to the casual observer, but down in the thick of the battle, you know. You know it's coming. Maybe not in the next minute, but in the next ten minutes, and the ten minutes after that, definitely. It's coming.

And now, with just over a quarter of the match left, it does come. Ken Owens rips like a fiend at a ruck and the ball squirts loose. Justin pounces, scooping it off his toes, and out it goes through the hands: Phillsy, Foxy, Cuthie haring down the right-hand touchline as the crowd rise as one. Brown's after him, but Cuthie's got the angle and the pace, and this time Brown misses the tap tackle and slaps his hands on the turf in despair as Cuthie goes over in the corner. It's 17–3. Bedlam.

Pence misses the conversion. England have a penalty which Farrell slides wide. Gethin comes off, which means I'm captain for the last 20 minutes or so, not that I have to do anything other than keep playing my game.

Jamie bashes through. Foxy skips a couple of tackles. We set up camp on the England 22. The forwards bash it up. I roll Dan Cole out of a ruck to give Phillsy clean ball, and he fires it back to Dan in the pocket. Drop goal, sweet as you like.

Now it's 20–3.

England kick off and knock on. Walsh plays advantage. Toby comes off the back of the ruck. He steps Tom Wood, then Geoff Parling, then Mako Vunipola – absurdly quick feet for a forward, but then again Toby's such a gifted all-round player that it's faintly ridiculous. Parling and Cole take him down. I'm right behind him, ready to pile in as the first man into the ruck, when I see something.

They've got no one sweeping.

They've got Dylan Hartley to the left and Danny Care to the right, but at the back of the ruck, where there should always be a man, there's no one.

I scoop the ball up and burst through the middle. Care tries to get to me but I fend him off with ease, and now I'm running free and the crowd roar is like a tsunami at my back. I look right, then left. The speed and suddenness of my burst has taken even my team-mates by surprise. All I can see are seven white shirts, some muddied and dirty and others still pristine, scrambling back behind me.

Ten metres. Twenty. Run, Forrest. Run.

Farrell's up ahead, waiting for me. Step him, but which way? Left or right? By the time I've made up my mind I'm on him, so it's the old Maori sidestep: bash straight through him. He goes high. Too high. I half-shrug him off and keep going a few more paces with him clinging onto my neck until Tom Croft arrives to help Farrell bring me down.

Alun Wyn and Bomb come piling in. Phillsy fires it out fast while England are still scrambling. The backs running from deep, hitting the line at pace, using the extra men well. Dan to Pence. Pence to Jamie, with Justin on his shoulder. Jamie commits the man and feeds Justin. Justin with Cuthie outside him and Mike Brown trying to cover both of them. Justin drawing Brown, shaping to pass, throwing the dummy and keeping on. Brown twisting desperately to follow the ball. Barritt half-catching Justin, just enough to slow him down and let Brown make the tackle second time round, but Cuthie's still on Justin's shoulder and he takes the pass to go in untouched. Second try, same corner as before.

Still on my hands and knees 40 metres away, I punch the ground as hard as I can in happiness.

Game, set, match, championship.

Before the trophy presentation, they turn out all the lights in the stadium. For a moment it's pitch black: then a spotlight comes on, shining on the podium.

The announcer calls us forward one by one, and every name is greeted by a huge cheer. After all the strife I've been through, to hear an entire stadium roaring their heads off at my name is the far side of amazing. I stand on the podium with all the other boys. This time last year, I was lifting the trophy with my one working arm while not really feeling I'd been a part of it all.

This time I do, even though – maybe especially because – I'm not captain. I did the first game and the last quarter of this one, but Ryan did three and Gethin started this one. I let them lift the trophy together and I honestly couldn't care less. We've won, that's all that matters. We've won in a match that none of us, and none of the spectators, will ever forget.

After the presentation, I walk round the field. Not a single Welsh fan has left. I punch the air in triumph at the crowd, and three tiers of people punch the air in unison back at me. I feel like a rock star. I honestly can't remember being happier on a rugby pitch. Moments like this are what make it all worthwhile. All the bad times, the injuries, the insults, the self-doubt, the pressure, the negativity – I can survive them all for moments like this. They can never take this moment away from me. Never.

After a performance like that, and with the Six Nations all over, the Lions taboo – which has lasted all season – is finally broken. As we come back into the dressing-room, there's a man slapping us on the back and saying 'See you in Australia' to each of us in turn.

Who? Phillsy, of course. Who else?

LEADERSHIP 4: PERSPECTIVE

No leader can do it all himself. It doesn't matter how experienced they are, how intelligent, how prepared or how committed. Every leader needs input from others to allow them to make the best decisions possible. They need perspective, and they can only get that perspective by consulting others.

During my career, I was lucky enough to always have people around me whose judgement I trusted, both off and on the pitch. These people didn't just give me good advice; they gave me fresh and interesting viewpoints too, because their personalities, their experiences and their areas of expertise were different not just from mine but from each other's too.

Off the field, I rarely, if ever, took a big decision without consulting seven (that number again!) people: my mum and dad, my brother Ben and sister Holly, Rach, Andy and Derwyn. If that effectively made Andy and Derwyn part of my family, well, that's how I saw them, because that's how much I trusted them. Each one of these seven had my best interests at heart, but each one of them also came at things from a slightly different angle:

- Dad knew how much I loved the confrontational side of the game, how important it was for me to get my Anthrax head on: refuse to be denied.
- Mum knew my doubts and emotional trigger points, and also looked at things from a mum's point of view, always worrying that her little boy was going to hurt himself.
- Holly saw things as a big sister, protective but also practical.

- Ben and I not only had the twin thing going on, but as the Blues physio he understood better than anybody what was happening to my body, and how much it could and couldn't take.
- Rach would know how much something would affect me on a day-to-day basis. She was the one who had to live with me, after all!
- Andy would look at things from the point of view of my mentality: how would a decision fit in with my self-image and the values I had?
- Derwyn would see things from a commercial and career-management point of view: how would something affect my financial situation, my long-term goals and my reputation?

Between them, then, I had pretty much all the bases covered.

The same was true on the pitch. At any one time with Wales, there were probably five players in total who between them took command. The personnel would vary, though not by that much; we had such a settled squad for most of my international career that the same people were there year after year. Men like Alun Wyn, Gethin, Jamie, Ken, Foxy, and so on. These five or so would meet every Monday morning to discuss things. In some ways we were one big captain, if that makes sense.

Every one of these guys brought something different to the table. Gethin was, by a mile, the best player I played with at assessing things on the field. He would often say to me, 'Go to the ref and say this.' It might just be the way the opposition were infringing at the breakdown, but he was so sharp, and he was almost always right. It was like having a coach on the field.

Jamie, as defensive leader at centre, was great at spotting what the opposition were trying to do. Alun Wyn was an inspirational character in the dressing-room. Those kind of things. They were a nucleus on which I relied a lot. Some people think that the captain is set apart from the other players, but if I saw myself as anything by way of captaincy it was first among equals, and with guys like that we were all very equal.

And of course you don't just have to seek the counsel of senior people. Everyone's got an angle, and everyone can contribute. In a rugby team alone you've got, for example, the hooker at the coalface, the enforcer in the second row, the dynamism and intelligence of the half-backs, and the full-back with the wide vision of the game that's unfolding in front of him.

No one person has everything. I played against lots of great 7s in my career, but not one of them was remotely perfect. To demonstrate this, if I were building the perfect 7 I'd take a little bit from seven different 7s. I'd take Tipuric's aerobic capacity and handling skills, Pocock's strength over the ball, Hooper's speed, McCaw's spatial awareness and ability to play so close to the edge, Dusautoir's tackling, Louw's ball-carrying, and my own explosive power in the rucks and discipline when it came to not conceding penalties.

That would be a perfect 7. But even then a player like that couldn't exist, because when you add quality in one aspect then, beyond a certain point, you have to start taking away from others. You can't be as strong as Pocock and as much of a greyhound as

Tipuric; you can't be as quick as Hooper and hit rucks with my explosive power.

The challenge as a leader is therefore twofold. One, to gather in advice from different people, but be aware that some of it will be contradictory and that you'll have to know which to use and which to discard. That is easier said than done. Some of this is experience, but much of it also comes down to the leader's second challenge: to be yourself. Listen to others, but always be yourself.

Some of the clubs I played for early in my career used to have initiation ceremonies, and the more outlandish and vile the better; one even involved putting a hole in the bottom of a black bag taken from a public bin and drinking the contents. That wasn't just gross – it was dangerous.

As a teenager I'd get so drunk at some of these events that I'd have to be scraped off the floor. I didn't like doing this, but I was young and the other players were older and more experienced, so I went along with it for a while.

Then one day I just thought, *I'm not doing this anymore. I'm not drinking at these things.* I got the piss ripped and called a shit bloke, but I stood my ground: and when I did, there were always other people who'd join me and say, 'I'm not drinking either.' They'd seen me stand up for myself, and that made them want to do the same for themselves. And in the end most people respect you for that, no matter how much grief they might give you at the time.

Be true to yourself. If you're happy standing up in front of a roomful of people and knocking out great speeches, go for it, knock yourself out. I wasn't. I hated being the centre of attention;

I never wanted to play the big 'I Am' or be Billy Big Bollocks. You see captains bringing everyone into a huddle on the pitch before or after a match, and you know that nine times out of ten they're doing it to look good for the cameras. You can huddle in the privacy of the dressing-room just as easily. The only time I ever did that on the pitch was if the opposition were late coming out and I didn't want the boys to lose focus.

Perspective often means equilibrium. As my old mentor and mate Martyn Williams told me – and these are words whose wisdom I had cause to reflect on several times during my career – 'You're never as good as they say you are, and you're never as bad either.'

5

ETIHAD STADIUM, MELBOURNE

37.8166°S, 144.9475°E

Saturday, 29 June 2013. British and Irish Lions v Australia, Second Test

Liam Gill takes the ball into contact. I go to jackal on him. Rob Simmons comes piling in on me. The hit rocks me slightly, but I stay in position. A split second later Ben Mowen smashes in, and now I'm half off the ball with my head down by my left knee, and that leg's trapped and extended straight.

If I get another hit now, I'm in trouble. If Genia clears it and the ruck breaks up I'll be OK, but one more hit with my leg caught like this is going to put me in a whole world of pain.

And that's when James Slipper makes the third hit.

It's like someone's taken a butcher's knife and slammed it into the back of my leg. The pain is white hot and almost indescribable. I have a brief image of my hamstring being cut clean off the bone, as though I'm nothing more than a carcass hanging from a ceiling hook.

Two words go through my head. Get up. Get up. Get. Up.

Andy Farrell's words: 'Unless you're unconscious or your femur's snapped, you're never injured in defence. If you can stand, you can get in line.'

I push myself upright.

The British and Irish Lions: the most special, the most unique, the most important thing in rugby.

The Lions are different, in every way. They have no home ground, no permanent coaching staff or players. They play almost all their matches on the other side of the world from where their personnel are based: they go to South Africa, Australia and New Zealand in turn, a tiny invading army far from home. They take players from four nations who are deadly rivals at international level and demand that they play for each other rather than against each other. Their kit is a mish-mash that reflects and includes all four of those nations: Wales in the shirt, England in the shorts, Scotland and Ireland in the socks.

For all but two months every four years, the Lions don't even exist, not really; but for those two months they are like a returning comet, blazing brighter and hotter than anything else in the rugby firmament. Lions tours take place in the year after the Olympics, the year before the football World Cup, and equidistant between Rugby World Cups. A Lions tour is arguably the biggest sporting event of its year; only the Tour de France can rival it.

In many ways, the Lions shouldn't work. Putting together a side from scratch to take on one of the big three southern hemisphere nations is a tall order at the best of times. Now take a bunch of players who are coming off long seasons for club and country, and condense the time they have together down to a few weeks. Mission impossible? By most rational yardsticks it should be, and sometimes it is.

But there's a reason not just why players would sell their own grandmothers to be a Lion, but also why tens of thousands of fans spend their life savings to come on tour and follow the team, and why the southern hemisphere players regard facing the Lions as up there with the pinnacles of their own careers. The Lions are a romantic sporting adventure with a long and cherished history. When you become a Lion, you want not just to live up to that history but add some of your own too. When the Lions get it right, it's the best feeling in the world.

For pretty much as long as I've played rugby, I've wanted to be a Lion. I'm so proud to play for Wales, yet I feel myself British quite as much as I do Welsh. My father's entirely English – Warburton's a good Lancashire name (that's where the bread comes from) – and my mother's great-grandparents were from Scotland, as her maiden name, Kennedy, shows. If I delve deep enough, I'm sure I can find some Irish in the family tree top. Hence my obsession with the Lions.

Now all I have to do is get picked. Problem is, every other Home Nations player has exactly the same aim.

I haven't had any contact with Gats throughout the entire Six Nations campaign this year. He's come to a few training sessions, as he has done for all four home nations, but I didn't speak to him at those; I didn't want to look like a kiss-arse or make it awkward for him if he was thinking of not picking me.

As for the captaincy, I've honestly never considered myself in the running. Sure, Gats appointed me Welsh skipper, but that means nothing. I'm still young, and I've never been on a Lions tour. If you ask me, either for my opinion on who Gats will pick or for who I'd pick if it was up to me, it would be one of the two previous captains: Paulie (Paul O'Connell), who did it in 2009, or Drico (Brian O'Driscoll), who was skipper in 2005 and whose tour ended when his shoulder was dislocated after being spear-tackled 41 seconds into the first Test.

And people do ask me, again and again and again. Some days it seems as though every journalist I've ever met rings up to ask if I've heard anything yet. No, I say, I haven't, and that's the honest truth. What I don't say is the second bit: *even if I had, mate, I'd hardly be telling you.*

Dad rings and says the local bookies have stopped taking bets on me.

'Dad, I don't even know what that means.' I've never placed a bet in my life.

'They think you're such a dead cert that they'd have to pay out on every bet involving you, so they just don't accept those bets any more. Someone must have caught wind of something.'

'Well, if they have, they haven't told me.'

I know, of course, that there are people who'll know the decision maybe even before the designated captain does. The coaching staff who between them make that decision, of course. The commercial and social media teams, so they're primed to get the news out quickly and efficiently. People love knowing things. Any one of those people might mention it to their wives in bed, who in turn will tell a friend or two, who in turn will tell another friend, and before you know it the gossip's going round like wildfire. Right now, having inside and advance knowledge of the identity of the Lions captain is the holy grail of any rugby fan. If you know, you'd find it almost impossible to keep your mouth shut. No one will believe you once it comes out if you say, 'Ah, I knew all along.'

Saturday, 20 April. We lose 24–6 to the Scarlets in Llanelli. I'm put up for press duties afterwards. Do the journalists want to talk about the match? Do they heck.

'Sam, what do you think about the bookies suspending betting on you becoming Lions captain?'

'I can honestly say, on my mother's life, I have no inkling of anything. The players are often the last people to find out about these things, so I'll just keep my head down for the Blues. One minute it's O'Connell, the next minute it's O'Driscoll, the next minute it's myself. It's difficult from a player's point of view. The decision is completely out of my hands.'

'Do you even want to be captain?' It might sound a silly question, but it's not. It's no secret that I've been a reluctant captain for Wales, and in fact – the last 20 minutes against England aside – I haven't skippered the side in any of our last four matches.

'It's a no-brainer. It's the biggest honour for any player. It's mind-blowing when you think about it, to have that accolade. Everybody who has done it has been a legend and it's flattering to think you are in contention for it. I still don't see myself as one of those players, really. It's quite strange, especially at twenty-four. If somebody had told me when I was watching the last Lions tour that I could be in this situation as a potential candidate, I'd have laughed.'

Sunday, 21 April. Rach and I are round at Mum and Dad's. I'm recovering from last night's match, Mum's on the phone to a friend, Dad's on shift at Whitchurch Fire Station. My mobile's charging on the kitchen table.

Just a typical quiet Sunday afternoon.

My mobile rings. I pad over to it without much urgency. It's probably just a mate calling or something. I don't get there in time before it rings off. I look at the screen.

Missed Call: Gats.

That quiet Sunday afternoon's just gone straight out of the window. I haven't had a call from Gats for ages, and I know he must be calling in connection with the Lions. What I don't know is whether he's calling to offer me the captaincy, or to tell me why he's gone with someone else, or maybe even explain to me that I'm not in the squad at all.

I unplug my phone and run upstairs to my old bedroom, which my folks now use as a nursery for my little nephew Harrison when he visits. I shut the door and ring Gats back.

'Gats, it's Warby.'

'Hello, mate. How you feeling?'

'Good, thanks.'

'How was the match last night?'

'Ah, you know. Always disappointed to lose.'

Get on with it.

'How's your body feeling after it?'

'Never better.'

'Really?'

'Really.'

'Good.'

For the love of God, Gats, just get on with it. One way or the other, just tell me.

Silence. I don't say anything. Gats clears his throat.

'Do you want to be captain of the British and Irish Lions this summer?'

I just laugh, equal mixtures of relief and disbelief. 'You bet. Yes, of course, I do. What an honour.'

We quickly discuss how things will pan out from here on in – where I'll need to be and when, how it's absolutely imperative to keep things secret until the official announcement nine days from now – and then he rings off.

I run back down the stairs, punching the air in delight.

'I'm Lions captain!' I blurt out to Rach.

Mum's still on the phone. I type **I'm captain of the Lions! C U later. Bye** into my mobile and hold it up so she can see it. Her mouth falls open and she totally loses the thread of what she was saying.

'I'll call you back later,' she says to her friend, before hanging up and giving me a huge hug.

I ring Dad to tell him.

'Gats has just phoned up and told me I'm going to be Lions captain,' I say.

'Ah, great,' he says, but he doesn't exactly sound overjoyed. 'Brilliant. OK.'

'Dad, did you hear me right? I'm going to be Lions captain.'

'That's great, Sam. I'll give you a ring back in a few minutes.'

When he phones back, he's much more enthusiastic. 'Sam, that's unbelievable news.'

'It's amazing, isn't it? There've been so many people asking that …'

'Yeah, OK. I'll talk to you later.' And he hangs up again.

For a moment I'm baffled, then I twig what must be happening. His colleagues at the fire station love their rugby and have all been desperate to find out if I'm going to be captain. Dad simply can't let on to them why I'm phoning, so he has to play it cool until he can get to talk to me without being overheard; but pretty much the moment he phones back someone walks into the room, so he has to act all nonchalant again. I know he must be as thrilled as Mum and Rach are.

The three of them are the only ones I tell. I can't tell anyone with any connection to rugby, so that rules out even Ben, who's a physio for the Dragons, Andy and Derwyn. It's not that they'd tell people off their own bat – I trust them with my life – but they could easily give it away accidentally by their reactions if people press them on it.

Wednesday, 24 April. Derwyn comes round for a catch-up.

'No word about the captaincy yet?' he asks.

'Not a dicky bird.'

Thursday, 25 April. The Cardiff Blues boys are still asking whether I know anything. I feel bad at having to lie to them, but I've no choice. Imagine if I let it slip, a couple of the boys went to put money on me, and all that came out. I'd be in serious trouble, even if I hadn't made any money myself, and rightly so.

I certainly can't tell the front-row players, as they'd doubtless be dense enough to go to the Paddy Power right across the road from the Arms Park.

'Ten grand on Warby to be Lions captain, please.'

'Right you are, sir. Hold on a moment while I call the cops.'

Friday, 26 April. The announcement's due next Tuesday. I really have to let Derwyn know before then. I ring him and tell him.

'Mate, that's great news,' he says. 'I'm delighted.' He pauses. 'Did you know when I came to see you a couple of days ago?'

'No. I didn't.' I'm glad he can't see my face.

I do decide to tell Andy after all, though. I guess it's because he has fewer direct contacts in the rugby world than Derwyn so I worry less. He'll have less opportunity to give the game away.

Monday, 29 April. I'm taken up to Syon Park in London in an unmarked Range Rover – no Lions branding on the side, of course, and they don't want me to drive my own car in case people recognise the number plate. The Lions team are so paranoid about leaks that they don't even let me come in the main entrance. Instead, I'm escorted in through the delivery entrance, through the kitchens and laundry, and up to my room via a back way. All very James Bond. I bet 007 would have made a decent openside, and not just because of the number. Tricks of the trade, skirting close to the edge of the law, not afraid to get hurt …

What with this and the secret cut-throughs I've discovered at the Vale to avoid the fans on match day, I should start compiling a list. Not so much *Warby's Winning Ways* as *Warby's Wormy Ways*: a guide to hidden passages in hotels throughout the rugby-playing world. Niche, perhaps, but there must be a market for it somewhere.

I have to stay in my room all the rest of the afternoon and evening. There's a revolving door of people coming to see me: press officers, photographers, social media operators and so on. I have to have dinner in my room and stay off social media in case my location comes up – though even that causes gossip in itself, with lots of people tweeting things about how suspiciously quiet I'm being just before the Lions announcement.

Tuesday, 30 April. Just before the announcement, I'm smuggled back down through the kitchen and into the back of the conference room. The place is packed.

Gats stands up and tells the world that I'm Lions captain. I walk up to the stage. TV lights and applause.

This is huge. This is so much bigger than the World Cup was.

I'm the only one who already knows I'm in the squad. With national teams, there are texts and emails sent before the news goes to the press. Not with the Lions. This is another subtle reminder that the Lions are different. The players find out the same way everyone else does, by watching the announcement live on Sky Sports. They gather with their families and friends at home, or with their team-mates at their clubs, and their joy (and their despair, if they haven't made it) is spontaneous and visible.

For weeks, perhaps months, players, fans and reporters alike have been picking their Lions squads, tweaking their selections after every round of the Six Nations to take account of form and injury: who's playing themselves in, who's playing themselves out? But only one selection matters, and it's this one.

Sky Sports' Alex Payne interviews me on stage. 'It's going to be new for me,' I say. 'I'm going to learn along the way. It's an experience that I just can't wait to get under way now. I'm always the ultimate optimist. I'll go out there with the intention to win every match. That'll be the great challenge for the players, as no other Lions team has done that.'

There are 10 matches, including three Tests. I mean every word of what I said, but I also know that Lions tours are first and foremost about the Test series. The provincial games are all well and good, but if you lose a couple because you're trying out new combinations or because you're using your midweek team, so be it. It's not even about winning an individual Test. It's about winning at least two of them, so you win the series. The Tests are the climax of everything that has gone before.

Gats talks about that moment in the England match when referee Steve Walsh pinged me for dragging at a ruck. 'Walsh allowed Sam to go to him three times to question that decision, to get some clarification. Now, if you know Steve Walsh, he doesn't allow that from anybody. Sam wasn't captain that day and you've got to be pretty special to be able to do that, because knowing Steve Walsh, he normally gives it the old "get away!"

'It was a big signal to me that either referees had been talking or it was about respect. There are only two or three players in the world that referees would allow to do that. It's the ability Sam has to communicate with referees; and when I saw that against England, it really stuck in my mind that this guy could do a job for us and potentially have a positive influence on the game with his relationship with referees.'

Thursday, 2 May. I'm with Derwyn.

'You know when I came to see you last week and asked if you were captain?'

'Yes. And I did know, and I should have told you.'

He smiles and winks. 'Thing is, Sam, I knew too.'

'You did?'

'I did. And I didn't put any pressure on you to tell me. I know it must have been a hell of a secret to carry.'

'How did you know?'

He smiles again. 'I'm a very resourceful man.'

Friday, 3 May. Phil Davies, coach of the Blues, asks Pence and me to go to Heath Hospital in Cardiff. There's a seriously ill lad in there who's a mad keen rugby fan. He loves the Blues, he loves Wales, and Pence and I are his favourite players.

This lad's in a bad way. He's missing a couple of limbs, his face is misshapen by all the tumours on it, and he can't speak. It's only three miles from my house to the hospital, but the way his eyes light up when he sees us, I'd go 300 miles to see that look. We sign all the shirts and flags and balls he has, and chat to his mum and dad, and pose for photos. It's only half an hour or so out of our day, but we can see that we've made this lad's year, and it humbles both of us.

We walk out of the hospital in silence. It's a trite and easy thing to say, but that doesn't make it any less true: we take so much for granted, and we are so lucky.

Friday, 10 May. Phil Davies phones. That lad who Pence and I went to see last week has died. Thank God we went to see him and did what we could for him. I know it meant a lot to him, but it meant just as much to us.

Monday, 13 May. It's Messy Monday: when all the boys selected for the Lions gather at Syon Park to get our kit and suits, and to meet each other, the coaches and the sponsors. If watching the announcement live must have been like waiting for GCSE results, this is more like the first day back at school, full of banter but also apprehension. 'I can't believe how nervous I am!' George North says.

I thought I knew most of the squad already, but that's partly because there are more boys from Wales than from any other country. Now I realise that, apart from a quick post-match handshake here and there, I don't actually know that many of the others: a few of the Irish boys (Paulie, Jamie Heaslip and Sean O'Brien) and Manu Tuilagi, but that's pretty much it. And that seems to go for most blokes here. People tread carefully, sizing up each other's personalities without giving away too much of their own. It'll take time for everyone to relax.

Adidas are supplying the kit, and they've really gone to town. There are personalised boots, and a laser instrument measures the exact size of our calves and ankles to make recovery skins for us to wear on flights throughout the tour. The attention to detail is remarkable.

One by one, the management team stand up, introduce themselves and say a few words. I'm the only one of the players to do the same. I talk about the lad who Pence and I went to see in hospital, the lad who died only a few days ago.

'Imagine the joy we gave to that boy. If only I could have had the power to say to him: "You'll be OK. You'll play for the Lions one day." That's what we've got. We're doing something that so many people would love to do. This is our opportunity. Let's not waste it.'

Andy and I go up into the woods near my home in Rhiwbina. There's a bench up there that I call my 'happy place'. I come here on my own or with the dogs, and I like to sit on the bench and just reflect. It overlooks the whole of Cardiff and the bay, and I can see the Millennium Stadium from here. It's only about five miles between the two places, but the contrast between the nerves and emotion of a match day and the tranquillity of this bench up in the woods is enormous.

'There'll be plenty of times on tour when you'll need to switch off,' Andy says. 'And it'll be hard with so much going on. So this is an exercise to help you with that. Close your eyes, do the controlled breathing techniques we've practised so often, and relax. Clear your mind completely. Tell me when the first thing comes into your head.'

I do what he says, but it's only about five seconds until I think of something and blurt it out. He makes me try it again, and again, and again. Gradually I let myself take in the peace and calm of the woods around me: listening to the birdsong, feeling the breeze on my face, smelling the earth. It's not long until I'm managing a couple of minutes, my mind totally empty and my body relaxed.

I take a photo of the view, and Andy takes a picture of me standing and looking out over it. 'Keep these on your phone,' Andy says. 'Whenever you feel under stress on tour, look at these photos and take yourself back here.'

*   *   *

I drop my dog Gus off at Mum and Dad's and say goodbye to him.

Later that day, I'm driving past when I have a sudden thought: I should say goodbye to Gus again. So I go in and give him another hug.

Mum doesn't bat an eyelid. She's quite used to how soppy I am around dogs.

I quickly realise that something I thought might be a problem – getting the boys to overcome their national rivalries – isn't going to be an issue at all. Everybody's so thrilled to be here in the Lions camp, so determined to make the most of the opportunity, that they just put aside anything which might hinder that.

Maybe that's not too surprising. There are four regional teams in Wales – the Blues, the Dragons, the Ospreys and the Scarlets – and the rivalries between them are fierce, but when boys from those teams come together for Wales, there are never any problems. The same principle applies here. For four regions, read four nations. As far as Home Nations rugby's concerned, the players selected for the Lions are the best of the best, and we all want to prove that.

Jamie Roberts puts it well. 'It's about handling pressure well, it's about complete enjoyment, getting along with everyone on the tour, taking every opportunity that comes your way and giving your all to the shirt. If you don't give your all, you are doing an injustice to all those that have been selected before you.'

* * *

No one knows the Lions better than Geech – Sir Ian McGeechan – who's been on seven tours, five as a coach (including four as head coach) and two as a player. No wonder he called his autobiography *Lion Man*.

'The crucial thing about the Lions,' Geech says, 'is that every tour is different. Every time a tour party is announced, that group of players has no identity, character or meaning until they actually meet up. Some tours might have a rump of players who were on the previous tour, but generally every tour is different because the players are always different. It is not one team that on the field looks the same or plays the same. It is a team that on its day creates a very unique sort of character and characteristics. It becomes distinguished and identified by the year it took place: "the 1974 Lions" or "the 1989 Lions", or the like.'

We are the 2013 Lions, and this is our chance to make our year a vintage one.

All Lions tours come with pressure, but this one more than most. It's been 16 years since the Lions last won a series, the 1997 tour to South Africa. Since then, the Lions have undertaken a complete southern hemisphere cycle – Australia in 2001, New Zealand in 2005 and South Africa in 2009 – and lost the lot.

Even that doesn't tell the whole story. Of the nine Tests over those three tours, the Lions lost seven in a row and won just two: the first one in Australia and the last one in South Africa. But the latter was only after the series had been lost, which means that of those nine Tests the Lions won only one when the series in question was still live.

It's not quite true to say that the Lions' survival rests on us winning this series – the amount of money the Lions generate shows that the concept is still very much a viable one – but if we lose again, especially with what already looks like a very tricky tour to New Zealand in four years' time, then people will start to question whether the Lions still have a place in an increasingly crowded international calendar. I don't want to be the captain who history shows presided over the beginning of the end.

Winning isn't just important for the Lions as a whole, of course. It's important for each and every player as an individual too. It reminds me of the conversations I had in New Zealand during the World Cup with locals who said, in all seriousness, that they wouldn't consider McCaw a true great until he'd won the World Cup.

The same applies here. For Drico, this is his fourth tour, and he's yet to win one; the previous three have comprised that complete cycle of southern hemisphere losses. 'It's about time I won one of these,' he says. 'I've certainly had enough cracks at it. Until you win a series, it's difficult to place yourself in that elite group of great Lions players. You've got to win a series to be properly remembered.

'I've talked to Matt Dawson about that dummy over-the-head pass that secured the first Test win in South Africa in 1997. How many times have people spoken to Scott Gibbs about his big hit on Os du Randt in Durban? These moments are timeless – but they're only timeless because of the victory that followed. To be considered a great and a custodian of Lions rugby you have to achieve that success. It's not enough to produce one-off performances or be nearly men. I'm definitely not going to be involved in the next World Cup, so this is my last big moment in rugby.'

All successful Lions tours have two things in common. First, that the guys selected are not just good players – that's taken for granted – but also good tourists. If boys go off reservation or turn negative, usually because they haven't made the Test team, that can cause disharmony. Every second counts on a Lions tour, for good and for bad. Faith and trust are just as important as skill and fitness. Out on tour, thousands of miles from home, all you have is each other.

Second, that everyone feels they have a fair crack of the whip in pressing their claims for Test selection. Clearly the coaches have a Test team in mind even before we leave Heathrow, but that team may change, perhaps drastically, depending on how people play on tour.

On the 1997 tour, Geech and Jim Telfer picked purely on form; how many pundits would have had Tom Smith and Paul Wallace in the front row, or Jeremy Davidson at lock? But they were the best players in those positions on tour, and so they were picked (and, not coincidentally, helped win the series).

Conversely, the 2005 New Zealand tour saw Sir Clive Woodward widely criticised for relying too heavily on the English players he'd coached to the World Cup two years earlier, even though many of them were not playing as well either as they had then or as some of the other boys in the squad. The Lions lost that series 3–0.

Gats has emphasised time and again that this is a squad more like the first of those examples, one where everyone can compete for a Test starting place. That's the best way to be, putting everyone on edge in training. Watching the boys working on weights and fitness, you can tell people have lifted it from international level. The bar has been raised, quite literally.

The strength and conditioning guys say that they're looking for our KPIs, our key performance indicators, to be between eight and ten metres per minute higher than usual. Over the course of a match, that means we'll be covering half a mile extra. It might not sound a lot, but trust me, it is.

Saturday, 1 June. We batter the Barbarians 59–8 in Hong Kong, a match in which the weather conditions – high 30s and 95 per cent humidity – prove far tougher opposition than the guys we're playing against. We have to have breaks midway through each half so the players can take on liquid and cool themselves in front of giant fans spraying water droplets.

The strength and conditioning coaches say the stopover will help with the jetlag, and they talk about the fitness benefits of working our bodies in such extreme conditions, but we all know the game is primarily a money-spinning exercise – after all, our shirt sponsor is the Hong Kong and Shanghai Banking Corporation. And fair enough. The Lions wouldn't be viable without large-scale commercial backing, and we're all used to having to fulfil sponsor commitments.

I don't play, as I'm still recovering from my knock, but even so it's nice to get some kind of revenge for the Barbarians defeat two years ago. Some of the Barbarians players here today seem to be sweating out neat alcohol, if the smell's anything to go by, so their preparation methods clearly haven't changed too much.

Sunday, 2 June. We're flying from Hong Kong to Perth, but there's a slight problem. There's one less business-class seat available than there are players, which means someone will have to travel economy. I volunteer to do it myself – it would be a small way of emphasising that I really don't see myself as better than or different from any of the other boys – but I'm carrying a slight knock to my knee, and the physios say I need the extra space in business to stretch out and aid my recovery.

Gats decides to have some fun. At the squad meeting before we leave for the airport, he gives it some *X Factor*-style suspense, whittling the candidates down bit by bit. First he rules out anybody playing in the match against Western Force on Wednesday. Then he rules out any of the second rows, as they're too tall. Then he rules out anyone like me who's even slightly injured. Finally, we realise there's only one guy left – Hibbs.

Everyone gives Hibbs some good-natured abuse, and being Hibbs he gives it back with interest. Every tour needs a character like Hibbs: a joker, someone always up for a laugh, a character on and off the pitch. In four years' time in New Zealand, Kyle Sinckler will take on this role. Maybe it's a front-row thing. But as Hibbs, grumbling away and giving us the finger, turns right at the entrance to the plane while we all turn left, you don't have to be Sigmund Freud to know that guys like him on tour are worth their weight in gold.

Wednesday, 5 June. Western Force don't provide any more opposition than the Barbarians had. We beat them 69–17. It's always hard to get a decent handle on how well the boys are playing when you have walkovers like this, but there are a lot of guys out there who look very good indeed. Pence kicks 11 from 11, more than half of those from out on the touchline. Drico and Manu play well together in the centre, George and Mako Vunipola look like seasoned veterans rather than Lions rookies, and I'm going to have to work hard to get a Test spot ahead of Sean O'Brien on this form.

We all know that sterner tests await, not just the Tests themselves but matches against the better Super Rugby franchises, and we can't wait for them, even if the Wallaby management has ensured we won't face some key players until the Tests themselves. 'We'd like to be playing against stronger sides,' Gats says. 'If we can't, then we're going to have to replicate that at training. It's something we learned from 2009. We arrived at the first Test thinking we were in good nick and found it was a big step up. We won't get caught this time.'

The scale of a Lions tour has to be seen to be believed. There are 40 players and 40 support staff, and no stone is left unturned.

There's an entire team of staff we never see, as they're always either ahead of or behind us, making sure everything's in place at the next venue, packing things up at the last one once we've left. We each have five bags of stuff, and whenever we get to a new hotel room they're already laid out neatly for us. We get fed five times a day. The social media guys are forever churning out content to help us connect with the fans in the country with us and with the public back home.

The video analysts in particular are amazing. I'm not sure they ever sleep; they're already there when we come down to breakfast each morning, and they're still working when we turn in for the night. They send clips to our phones that show our opposite number in the next match we'll play; in my case, the carries he's made, the tackles he's executed, the ruck cleanouts he's done.

Look, these clips tell you, here's where he competes and doesn't compete, these are the patterns to his play, these are his strengths you need to counter, these are his weaknesses that you might be able to exploit. You might not get the chance in the game itself, of course, but if you do then you have to take that chance quicker than thought itself.

After our own training sessions, clips are available within three hours, with the coaches talking over the footage, explaining which parts were successful and which need more work. Then there are the PDF documents on the referees, outlining the number of penalties they give and the percentage of each specific offence within those penalties.

If a ref gives a high proportion of penalties for not rolling away, for example, then come the game I can point out to him that the opposition aren't rolling away, knowing that he's hot on that anyway. Probable result: he pings them a few times and I look like I know what I'm talking about.

Yes, every club and national team runs versions of all this stuff. You won't find a professional outfit these days that doesn't have nutritionists, video analysts and the like. But not to this extent, not really. With the Lions, everything is bigger, better, slicker and quicker.

Saturday, 8 June. Queensland Reds, Brisbane. Third match in, but my first runout; I didn't play in either Hong Kong or Perth, and I'm choking to get involved. When you haven't played you do feel out of the loop slightly, no matter how much you say that you don't. But I know I don't need too much game time to prove myself for Test selection, and I also know that after a tough season, rest is just as important as anything else. Missing the first two games won't have harmed my chances of making it through the tour; quite the opposite, in fact. Not that I can say any of this publicly, of course.

Every Lions player gets a cap number. The plaque above my spot in the changing room here at the Suncorp says: 'Sam Warburton. 800.' An easy number to remember.

We want the Reds to give us a good game, and they certainly do that, even without their seven Wallaby squad members. They come at us hard and fast right from the off, and take the lead when Luke Morahan snaffles a Faz kick, spins away from Cuthie, surges past Ben Youngs, fends me off, chips Stuart Hogg and wins the race to touch down. Seventy solo metres from start to finish – a brilliant try that justifiably has the crowd on their feet.

We gradually assert ourselves. Ben snaffles the ball from the back of their scrum to score from close range, and then George beats four men in a 50-metre run before passing it out to me. I step the first man and think I'm in, but then two defenders scrag me just short of the line. We turn round 16–7 up, and though they score another try, we hold our nerve and kick our points to win 22–12.

It's a good win against tough opposition, and we've learned more from that game than from the previous two combined. For my part, at least I can say I'm a proper Lion. But that's not enough. It won't be enough until I take that 7 jersey into the Test matches. Oh, I'd take a minute of a midweek Lions game up country over playing for Wales, but for me it's always been the Tests above all else. It won't be enough until I start those Tests with that number on my back, and finish them as the victor.

Tuesday, 11 June. We play a combined New South Wales and Queensland county side, and it's a complete mismatch. They're part-timers – students, engineers, removal men and plumbers among them – and they're not nearly fit or strong enough to cope. It's more or less a semi-opposed training run. In fact, most of the training sessions are tougher than this game, because our skill levels are so high.

The boys run in ten tries in a 64–0 victory, and perhaps we could and should get our score up to near the century mark. Justin in particular plays well. Perhaps a few months ago this would have worried me in terms of thinking about my own place, but I'm in a much better mental space now. It's good that he – and Sean, for that matter – are playing so well, as it forces me to up my game still further.

And if everyone on tour does that, then we'll be raring to go once the Test series starts.

Hibbs is in charge of fines, and when Gats is 30 seconds late for a meeting, Hibbs makes him roll the big fluffy dice that we use for forfeits.

Gats rolls a four. *Make your own way back from training. You may not carry either money or a phone. You have to walk if need be.*

Gats has only just recovered from breaking both heels when falling off the roof of his house in New Zealand. But Hibbs shows no mercy. He's been waiting since that flight from Hong Kong to Perth to get his own back on Gats. He's also probably the only person in the whole squad with the bottle to do this.

At least if Tom Youngs starts the Tests ahead of me I'll know why, Hibbs says.

Saturday, 15 June. For the second Saturday in a row I'm in the team, this time against the New South Wales Waratahs. The first Test's in a week's time, and there's only one more match between now and then, so this team is looking very much like the one that will probably start that first Test.

The Waratahs are a good side. This close to the Test series, we've got to beat them and beat them well. We've got to put down a marker: *we've beaten the joke sides you've offered up, and we've beaten the good ones too. We're here, and we mean business.* 'In this country,' Gats says, 'you need a strut, a swagger. That's what they respect.'

We don't just beat the Waratahs. We wallop them. We boss the show up front, and when they put in some cheap shots we don't retaliate. We score five tries, with Pence bagging two of them plus eight kicks for a personal haul of 30 points; as one report says, Pence 'is playing like JPR Williams, Gerald Davies and Jonny Wilkinson rolled into one'.

Foxy plays out of his skin, winning man of the match and attracting praise from a bloke who knows a bit about playing at outside centre. 'Man, how good was Jonathan Davies?' says Drico. The only downside is that Jamie Roberts hobbles off with 13 minutes left having done his hamstring.

Dave Dennis, the Waratahs' captain, seeks me out afterwards. 'If you play like that again next week,' he says, 'the Wallabies will struggle to compete.' He's a good bloke and it's a nice thing to say. It gives me confidence that we're heading in the right direction.

Tuesday, 18 June. We're playing the ACT Brumbies in Canberra. It's our last game before the Test series, and we lose it.

Yes, it's close: only two points in it, 14–12. Yes, none of the guys likely to start on Saturday are involved. Yes, both centres and both wings (Barritt, Billy Twelvetrees, Christian Wade and Shane Williams) are injury call-ups who've only just arrived in Australia. And yes, Gats said he'd swap a defeat here for victory on Saturday. The last time the Lions lost to a provincial side was against Northern Transvaal in 1997, and they came back from that to win the series.

But a loss is still a loss. And at this stage of the tour, a loss can be more than a loss. It can derail momentum and sap confidence. The boys out there tonight looked tired and a little flat – if nothing else, the travel schedule's been pretty hectic: Hong Kong, Perth, Brisbane, Newcastle, Sydney, Canberra – and at one stage they were 14–3 down. They don't even score a try, the first time that's happened in a Lions match since the final Test in New Zealand eight years ago.

It's important to salvage this right now rather than let it fester. The boys who weren't playing pile into the changing-room to offer condolences and try to pick the spirits up, but the room's got a slightly weird design – each player has more or less an individual cubicle rather than just a marked space on a bench – which makes it hard to get everyone together.

I'm just thinking about what I should say when Geoff Parling gets up.

'F*** what's just happened,' he says. 'It was bollocks, but it's gone and we can't change it. We tried our best. Shit happens. Crack on. Now it's up to us to help the Test team so they can do a job on the Wallabies on Saturday.'

It's not just what he says but the way he says it. Instantly, the mood's transformed. Whatever I'd been about to say I keep to myself. I'd be jumping in on the back of him and just saying something for the sake of it. Geoff has said it all, and it's another example of every good team needing leaders in multiple positions.

In fact, given the way he is both on and off the field throughout the tour, Geoff would have made a great Lions captain himself.

Wednesday, 19 June. The team for the first Test is announced. No matter how much you prepare for this, no matter how few surprises there are in selection – and most players are pretty good at working out where in the pecking order they stand – this is always a divisive moment. Up until now, the tour has been about players competing for those coveted Test match jerseys, and no decisions have been set in stone. Now they have, and half the party's missed out.

Most of those who miss the cut aren't used to it; they're first choice for their country, let alone their club. There's no way of soft-soaping that, even if you wanted to. Yes, there are three Tests and yes, things can change – form and injury mean that the team that starts the first Test is very rarely the one that starts the third – but right now the final game seems a long way off, whether you've made it or you haven't.

The training session immediately afterwards is the most savage one we've had yet. Not in terms of the coaches beasting us – they keep it short and sharp, with the Test only three days away – but in terms of the passion and frustration that all the boys bring to it. Those who've made the Test 23 are determined to show they deserve it; those who haven't are royally pissed off and determined to show the coaches they've made a mistake. The intensity leads to mistakes.

The coaches don't seem that bothered. It's clear they've seen this kind of thing before, and in fact the only thing that would worry them was if it wasn't like this.

Thursday, 20 June. With yesterday's aggro now out of everybody's systems, today's training session is as slick as yesterday's wasn't. We're looking good.

The fans are here in their thousands, thronging the bars on the banks of the Brisbane River and singing songs that remind the boys of home: 'Fields of Athenry', 'Swing Low', 'Flower of Scotland' and 'Cwm Rhondda'. On a national summer tour you get a few expats and diehards. This is light years away. Wherever you look, all you can see are red shirts.

Drico remembers the wall of red here 12 years ago, which so alarmed the Australian Rugby Union (ARU) that they spent $200,000 on green and gold T-shirts to give away in Melbourne and Sydney during the last two matches.

'That genuinely felt like a home game that day,' he says. 'We didn't even think that would be a possibility, and then we ran out and the ground was three-quarters red. The crowd have a huge role to play. They put extra pep in your step. It can be that little bit of extra incentive and inspiration you need to have the game of your life.'

Friday, 21 June. 'Red wall in D,' Andy Farrell says. 'Defence is the start of our attack. Make it positive. Don't just sit back and wait for them. Red wall in D, and f*** 'em up second phase.'

I'd have loved to have played with him in his heyday, He's a seriously hard bloke. You want to put your body on the line for him.

The coaches are calling on me, Paulie and Drico to lead: the current captain and the two previous ones. We need to show intelligence, energy and passion. There's a reason why we wear the Lions badge over our heart.

Geech hands us our jerseys, one by one. 'The jersey will come alive,' he says. 'It will demand more from you, as it has demanded more from all the others who have ever worn it. It's the most personal jersey you can wear, as it asks different things of you. It reflects your character.'

I'm last up to collect mine. As I walk to the front, I catch a glimpse of Jamie Heaslip. He's looking down at his jersey and stroking the badge softly.

Rala, the baggage man who's one of the Lions' real characters – 'My door's always open to you, 24 hours a day, except when it's closed' – asks me whether I want to give the jersey back to him to put in the changing-room tomorrow as usual, or whether I want to keep it with me and bring it to the game myself.

'No one's taking this from me,' I say.

I go back up to my room and put the shirt on my bed, face down so the number 7 is staring up at me, just like it had on the replica jersey I'd been given by my parents when I was 15. I remember putting that jersey away, vowing that the next time I wore it would be for real.

Now it is. It's almost as though I willed it into being, the replica shirt becoming the real one. In between the two lie years of sacrifice and hardship, of relentless self-improvement and occasional self-doubt, of refusing to be denied.

I leave the shirt on my bed and go to leave the room and join the others; but before I open the door, I go back to the bed to have another look. This beautiful, precious, priceless shirt.

I go to the door for a second time, and again I go back to look at the shirt.

Only on my third attempt do I manage to leave the room.

Geech's words.

What is a Test-match animal? Well, he is never prepared to be second. He knows what is required, and he does it again and again and again, and he does it in such a physical, determined and focused way that he is never going to be beaten. His instinct is just that little bit more ruthless than others'.

You can be a good international player, but what a Lions Test does is find out something more about a player. It is about that animal instinct. He is there not just for survival but also for control. He has an instinct to do the right thing that makes a difference. It is not in every international rugby player, but it is in every successful Lion.

It is about playing on the edge, but with intelligence and awareness. It's a combination of execution and decision-making. You can have all the skills and techniques from training. You can build experience from playing. But the instinct to do the right thing at the right time is inside you – that's the difference. To have that animal bravery, to know what you are doing is probably stupid, but to do it anyway with the conviction that it will tilt a game, is a special gift.

Saturday, 22 June. Brisbane. A sign on the wall. IF YOU DON'T TAKE A CHANCE THEN YOU DON'T STAND A CHANCE.

'Let's go into their house and smash them up,' Gats says.

In the changing-room. Rala's table piled with boxes full of everything we need: tape, scissors, studs, strapping, cotton pads, energy drinks, protein bars. Gathering the boys around me. I'm in the zone now, and my blood's up. Looking each man in the eye, knowing that they'll do what it takes. 'If they're into you, you f***ing pile into 'em,' I shout. 'Every single collision. Get up off the floor, work f***ing hard for your team-mates.'

Walls of red in the Suncorp, just like there'd been 12 years ago when Drico scored his famous try.

The match starts with a bang, almost literally. There's less than a minute gone when Christian Leali'ifano goes to tackle Foxy and knocks himself out on Foxy's hip. Foxy sees it immediately and calls for play to be stopped. You don't want to see anyone go off so early in a match, and it's a relief to both sides when Leali'ifano gives a thumbs-up as he's stretchered from the pitch.

Twelve minutes gone. Australia have a penalty deep in their own territory. Their scrum-half Will Genia has the ball. He's their danger man, the one we need to watch. He's not big, but his power-to-weight ratio's insane: he can bench double his own bodyweight. He ran Wales ragged at times last summer. He's got pace, he's got an eye for the gap and he links well with his back three. We need to keep him closed down, shepherd him back into the areas where we've got numbers and can smother him.

That's what we need to do. That's exactly what we fail to do.

Genia taps and goes, setting off on a mazy run. A dummy takes out Phillsy and Tom Croft, and now Genia's running at George and Pence. George is looking to the men outside: stay in or go out? Pence holds his position, trying to show Genia the outside; and as George and Pence converge on Genia, he pops a little grubber through to take them both out of the equation. Israel Folau scoops it up and runs round to score under the posts.

We can't say we weren't warned.

Just a little over ten minutes later, Berrick Barnes hoists it high to George just short of our 10-metre line. Two weeks ago George did his hammy, grade 1. To come back from that within two weeks is nothing short of amazing and shows how brilliant our physios are. This is another thing about the Lions: it's not just the players who are the best of the best, but all the staff too. Coming back from a hammy in two weeks is one thing, however. Putting that hammy under the stress of a Test match and seeing if it holds up is something else entirely.

'Off the pitch I'm not that confident,' George once said. 'But once I smell that whitewash, once I cross that line, I'm in a different zone. I find myself quite aggressive. Confident but not arrogant, and generally quite mad at everyone on the other team. I don't know what it is, but it's like they've done something.'

George is already moving when he takes the ball. I can see the intent in his eyes. I know what this means. When George is on, he's *on*.

He steps between two players, is half-caught by James O'Connor, stumbles, regains his balance, and keeps going. The Aussie cover is coming across, but George is too big and too quick for them. He skins Barnes with a step off his right foot and gestures at Genia as he goes in at the corner. It's the greatest individual try in Lions Test history, shading even Drico's effort here in 2001.

And George is still only 21. What were you doing aged 21? What was I doing aged 21? Coming on as a sub in Six Nations matches. Not scoring tries like that.

Together with a couple of Pence penalties, we're 13–7 up with just over five minutes to go until the break when Folau decides that anything George can do, he can do better. He beats Corbs (Alex Corbisiero), Johnny Sexton and Pence on his way to the tryline. Perhaps the rest of us should just stay in the shed at half-time and let George and Folau play one-on-one for the second 40.

At half-time it's 13–12.

The next score could be crucial, and it's ours. Johnny has the ball, Drico's decoy run takes O'Connor out of the picture, and Cuthie runs a beautiful angle back against the defence. Genia and Kurtley Beale both dive at him and both miss. Cuthie's mobbed by the subs in their orange tabards behind the in-goal area as he touches down. Lions 14, someone had written next to Cuthie's name back in the Vale during the Six Nations. Try-scoring Lions 14, as it turns out. Pence converts and that's 20–12: more than a score between the sides for the first time in the game.

No Aussie side knows when they're beaten, and this one's no exception. Two penalties bring them back to 20–18 just after the hour mark. Then they're pinged for being on the wrong side of a ruck, giving Pence a hard kick out on the right-hand side. Pence drills it through the posts as though the ball's laser-guided, making it 23–18.

Beale runs half the length of the pitch, jinking this way and that through the traffic. Their skipper James Horwill takes it on. I jackal him at the ruck. Roll away, referee Chris Pollock tells me. Australia take it into contact again, and this time they do get the penalty: 23–21.

This is a proper arm wrestle now: brutal, oscillating and enthralling. Huge efforts for tiny gains.

Two minutes to go and we're still holding out when the scrum wheels and breaks. Pollock blows instantly. Penalty to Australia, 45 metres out. It's difficult, but definitely kickable.

I can't believe it. My mind flashes back to Cardiff last autumn, and Sydney and Melbourne last summer: three games in a row when Australia took it from Wales in the dying seconds. *It can't be happening again, it just can't.* I look at the other Welsh boys on the pitch – Pence, Cuthie, Foxy, George, Hibbs and Lyds – and see that they're all thinking exactly the same.

Beale lines it up. *Here we go again.*

There are 20 seconds left on the clock when he starts his run-up.

In the last stride he plants his standing foot, but the ground's wet and chewed up from where the scrum's just been. Beale's foot slides from beneath him – shades of Hooky in the World Cup semi-final two years ago. Beale's already falling when he connects with the ball. For a moment I think it still might have the legs to make it, but then it starts to drop and it's clear that it's going to fall short and wide. Pence shepherds it over the deadball line and that's it.

We've won.

Not by much, and perhaps not totally convincingly, but neither of those matter. We've won, and for once a last-minute kick has gone our way and not Australia's. Defeats right at the death are so hard, psychologically. If we'd gone down like that again today, it would have been very hard to pick ourselves up again in time for Melbourne. I hug Pence and Cuthie. The Aussies are down on their knees, beaten and deflated. I know just how they're feeling, as they've made sure I've felt it several times myself.

Hooper, probably mindful of what happened between me and him in Cardiff last autumn, doesn't ask to swap shirts.

Sunday, 23 June. There's an enormous – and by enormous, I mean twice the size of a rugby pitch enormous – advert waiting for us in a field visible from the approach into Melbourne airport. ROOTING FOR THE WALLABIES, it says, above a picture of what Sportsbet, the firm responsible, describes as 'a wallaby hugging a lion from behind'.

So *that's* what they call it these days.

Tuesday, 25 June. The midweek team put 35 points past the Melbourne Rebels without reply. The win, and the manner of it, are important for two reasons. First, it's the last non-Test game of the tour, and keeping momentum ahead of the second Test is crucial. Second, there are places in the Test team up for grabs – Paulie's out for good with a fractured arm, Corbs will definitely miss Saturday with injury, and Phillsy's been struggling with a knock to his knee. Even without these problems, we didn't play well enough in Brisbane for the coaches not to consider making some unforced changes to go with the forced ones.

Lyds in particular has done his chances no harm at all. He was captain for the day, and his pre-match speech was like something out of a Vietnam war movie. On the pitch, he played like a man possessed, tackling everything that moved and quite a lot that didn't. I wouldn't be at all surprised to see him packing down on the opposite flank to me on Saturday. Assuming I make it, of course.

Wednesday, 26 June. Lyds is indeed in, with Tom Croft dropping to the bench. Tommy Bowe comes in for Cuthie at 14. The three injury changes are pretty much as expected: Mako for Corbs at loosehead, Geoff for Paulie in the second row, Ben for Phillsy at 9.

That's five of the starting XV – a third of the team – changed between the first and second Tests. When coaches say that Test spots are still up for grabs right until the end, those aren't idle words. It can and does happen, and it's up to every player to be ready to take their opportunities the moment they arrive.

This is the Lions, and it does special things to people. There's no way, for example, that you could play a club match with the intensity of Lyds's performance against the Rebels and then do it all over again in a Test four days later. But for the Lions, you do. You just do. You do anything. Your body finds a way to go beyond.

Thursday, 27 June. A Lions tour can be all-consuming when you're in the thick of it, so now and then it's good to get some perspective. I'm walking with Rach, George and his fiancée Becky (James, the GB track cyclist) around Melbourne, and we don't get recognised once. Not that we're complaining. It's nice just to be able to chill out without being stopped every five seconds for a selfie.

We see a big posse of Lions fans in the distance, but we're too far away for them to spot us. An Aussie woman sees us looking at the fans and comes up to us.

'Who are all those guys in the red shirts?' she asks.

'They're Lions fans,' I say.

'Lions? What's that? AFL?' Aussie Rules, to you and me.

'No. Rugby.'

'You mean league?'

'Union.'

She looks sceptical, as though union's a long way down the pecking order. Maybe she's right; in terms of player numbers, it's behind cricket, Rules, league and soccer.

'These Lions – where are they from?'

'Britain and Ireland.'

She shakes her head in good-natured bemusement at people flying halfway round the world to watch a game of union, and goes on her way.

Friday, 28 June. I see Mum and Dad. They wish me luck, but they seem a bit quiet and distracted, not quite their usual selves. I put it down to jetlag, nerves about tomorrow, or both. Besides, I'm beginning to gear myself up for tomorrow's match, so maybe I'm not quite as attentive to their moods as I could be.

Saturday, 29 June. Some of the locals might not have any idea who we are, but the Lions fans here in the Etihad do. They're so desperate for us to win that it seeps through even into the warm-up. As we go through our pre-match drills, I find myself blinking back tears.

The second Test in a three-match series is always a titanic one, just because of the maths. One side's fighting to stay in the series, the other's fighting to close it out and make the final Test redundant. 'We have to finish them off now,' Drico says. 'Not next week, when it'll be much harder. Now.'

But in some ways it's easier being 1–0 down than 1–0 up. At 1–0 down you have to go for it as though there's no tomorrow: it's shit or bust. At 1–0 up, though, if you're not careful you can find yourself being too cautious and conservative, trying to reduce risk rather than embrace it. Even at 1–0 up you have to play as though you're 1–0 down.

We certainly start that way, fast and furious. Noise and pressure, putting Genia in trouble and forcing Beale to clear hurriedly. *Up a level from last week*, that's our message to them. *Whatever time and space you had in Brisbane, you won't find them here.*

Hooper takes the ball into contact. I jackal for it. Me against three of them, but I'm still there and Craig Joubert pings

Hooper for holding on. Pence hits the bar with the penalty and Australia clear. We keep the pressure on, piling backs into a 13-man lineout, big driving mauls, kicks to the corner. Again Hooper takes it into contact, and again Mako and I wrestle it clear for another turnover. Eighty-five per cent of the first ten minutes is played in their half, and Pence's second penalty attempt goes over.

I'm playing hard and smart. I go to compete at one ruck, before seeing that there are enough bodies there already and backing off into the defensive line. James Horwill comes through and bashes into me. I take him down, go to jackal, slow the ball down enough for our line to get back in place. Beale, frustrated, tries the cross kick, but Folau knocks on. That was all our defence, soaking up their attack and forcing them to try the risky plays out wide.

Quarter of an hour gone, and they have a penalty. Leali'ifano slots it: 3–3.

I tackle Ben Alexander and jackal him. Beale and Adam Ashley-Cooper pile in on me, but I'm still there. I'm on my game today. They go round the short side and Kane Douglas knocks on, again because we've left them with no options and are making them snatch at their chances.

Joubert's not happy with the way Mako's scrummaging, and Leali'ifano does the rest. Now we trade penalties: 6–6, 9–6 to us, 9–9 when Lyds strays offside. We're on the attack just before half-time and force them to concede the penalty. Pence makes no mistake, and we go in 12–9 up.

There's nothing in this, just as there wasn't last week either; and just like last week, we know this is likely to go right down to the wire.

'Let's have the f***ing courage to see this out now,' Drico snaps.

Fifty minutes gone. I surge through. Drico has men outside, but Folau picks off his pass and suddenly Australia have the attack with men on the left. Douglas crashes through inside the 22, Mako and I bring him down, he spills it and Pence clears. This is end-to-end stuff. The crowd are loving it.

Into the last quarter. Drico flicks it through his legs to George. Folau grabs George's shirt. For a moment the two men grapple each other before George, still holding onto the ball, hoists Folau in a fireman's lift as though carrying a stroppy kid up the stairs to bed, and starts running upfield with Folau on his shoulder. I've seen George doing reps up and down steps with 100 kg barbells on his shoulders, so I know he has the outrageous strength to pull this off, but to have the audacity to do it to an opponent an hour into a draining Test match is something else entirely. The crowd go nuts.

We have a scrum. We drive them back. Penalty: 15–9.

We need more. We need to be at least a score plus a bit ahead.

Quarter of an hour left. Liam Gill takes it into contact. I go to jackal on him. Rob Simmons comes piling in on me. The hit rocks me slightly, but I stay in position. A split second later Ben Mowen smashes in, and now I'm half off the ball with my head down by my left knee, and that leg's trapped and extended straight.

If I get another hit now, I'm in trouble. If Genia clears it and the ruck breaks up I'll be OK, but one more hit with my leg caught like this is going to put me in a whole world of pain.

And that's when James Slipper makes the third hit.

It's like someone's taken a butcher's knife and slammed it into the back of my leg. The pain is white hot and almost indescribable. I have a brief image of my hamstring being cut clean off the bone, as though I'm nothing more than a carcass hanging from a ceiling hook.

Two words go through my head. *Get up. Get up. Get. Up.*

Andy Farrell's words: 'Unless you're unconscious or your femur's snapped, you're never injured in defence. If you can stand, you can get in line.'

I push myself to my feet. Even putting the tiniest bit of weight on my left leg feels like a lightning strike. I hop into the defensive line. Hooper comes through and I can't get to him. He's taken down and I fall to the ground.

Have to get up. Have to stay in D. I grit my teeth against my gumshield and ride another wave of pain as I stand up once more. Hobble to the side of the ruck, in the guard position. *This could be the last thing you ever do as a Lion, so make it good; defend the phases, do your job for the team.*

Pointing at Genia, shouting 'I've got 9.' Kidology, pure kidology. A toddler could get through me right now. *Please don't come down my channel.*

They spin it wide, Beale knocks on, the whistle goes, and I slump to the floor once more. It's been 55 seconds since Slipper hit me. It's felt like 55 years.

Lying on my back, looking up at the stadium lights. That's it for me. Tour over. I can try and kid myself that it's not that bad, but I know it is. This is not something I'm coming back from in a few days. Injury #11.

The medics come on. 'Don't even bother assessing me,' I say. 'Just get me off.'

'Stretcher's coming,' says head doctor James Robson.

'No way. I'm walking off.'

'That'll only make it worse.'

I almost smile. 'Doc, it's screwed anyway. Walking off won't make a difference.'

I struggle to my feet. I put one arm round James's shoulder and the other round Prav's, and together we make our slow and painful way off the pitch.

I don't know it at the time, but Clive Woodward is calling the 65 minutes I played 'the most outstanding performance I have ever seen from a Lion'.

But that doesn't matter. What matters is that we hold on for the win.

And the Aussies are coming. Even though we're six points up, they're making all the play. Ten minutes left when Folau, even though he has no space to work in, beats two players before Pence brings him down. Genia runs sideways, Stephen Moore straightens, Tom Croft makes the tackle. Genia cross kicks for Joe Tomane, and Tommy snaffles him.

Back they go for the penalty. Eight minutes left. They take the scrum, keep the pressure. There's a scrum cap on the ground, ripped clean off someone's head in the frenzy. The ball's coming quicker for the Aussies now. I so want to be back in there, slowing it down and eating up the minutes. But I can't even walk.

Genia marshalling his troops. Now going left, now going right. Folau comes short off 9 and Lyds chops him. Men crowding the narrow side. Pick and go, make the hard yards. Five metres out. Genia sends it left again, and now they have a man over and they have space. O'Connor runs the angle, delaying the pass, waiting for Drico to make the hit – and here's Ashley-Cooper on the cutback as Foxy and Tommy are caught going the wrong way on the drift, and Ashley-Cooper's sliding over for the try and the crowd are roaring with him.

Australia one point down with the conversion to come.

Leali'ifano ignores the charging defenders and nails the kick. Australia now a point up, 16–15. Three minutes for us to pull something out of the fire.

O'Connor clears from inside his 22, but Genia was outside the 22 when he made the pass, so we have the lineout near their line. Poor game management from the Wallabies – you wouldn't expect an amateur club side to make that mistake – but it just shows how fatigue and pressure can scramble the brains of even the best players in the world.

We have to secure ball off this lineout. *Have to.*

We don't. Gill does brilliantly to take the ball one-handed at the tail – he used to play American football, and it shows – and win the penalty.

The hooter: 80 mins. Next time the ball goes dead, the match will be over. We're on the attack. Joubert pings them for holding on, just inside our half. Too far out for Pence. We run it. Johnny takes it up to halfway. Conor Murray digs into the ruck and appeals to Joubert – they're holding on again. Again Joubert blows, and again he gives the penalty.

If we trusted our lineout we'd kick deep, but we don't. On halfway. With the angle, 53 metres. Right at the edge of Pence's range. He nods. He'll have a go.

We thought this would go down to the wire, and it has. For the second time in a week, a last-minute, long-range kick to win the match. In Brisbane it was them; in Melbourne it's us.

Pence tries to steal a metre or two. Joubert's having none of it.

Eighty-two minutes gone. Whatever happens, this is the last play of the game.

Sound and fury fading away. Just one man, one ball, one set of posts.

Pence hits it well. It's high, it's hanging …

… it's falling. It's falling. It hasn't got the legs.

Genia catches it and kicks it out. Horwill's in tears. Pence is on his knees, crouched over as though he's been hit in the solar plexus.

One-all. Echoes of 2001, the last time the Lions toured here. Both times, the Lions won in Brisbane and lost in Melbourne; both times, the Lions' openside was forced off before time in the second Test.

The Aussies won that series. They're not going to win this one.

'A tough, tough Test,' Gats says.

'As tough as they come,' adds Robbie Deans, the Aussie coach.

'At times,' Johnny (Sexton) says, 'it felt like we were just wishing for the game to finish rather than going after it.'

Hard to argue with any of that.

I see Mum and Dad in the stands.

'Gus has died,' they say. That's why they were so quiet yesterday: they'd just got a text from Ben telling them, and they didn't want to distract me before the Test. After they saw me they went out to dinner at the nearest Wagamama, and were both in such floods of tears that the waiter thought they must be going through a hideously traumatic divorce or something.

I remember going to say goodbye to Gus twice before I left. At some deep level I must have known that I wasn't going to see him again.

I hobble back to the changing-room. Doing my hamstring, losing the Test and now this: a triple-decker shit sandwich all in the space of half an hour. I slump in the corner and burst into tears.

'What's wrong, mate?' says Jamie Heaslip. 'It's only a hamstring.'

Sunday, 30 June. We go to do some recovery work in the sea at St Kilda. It's freezing, and we're all feeling pretty down.

There's a bunch of women in bikinis there, and they come over to chat. Our security guys aren't impressed. They think it's a set-up, and that somewhere in the dunes will be snappers with long lenses who'll get pictures of us – many of us married or with partners – chatting to women in bikinis when we've just lost a Test. A cheap trick, but no less effective for that.

'Back on the bus,' the security guys say. 'Now.'

The coaches protest. 'They haven't done enough time in the water yet.'

The security guys are ex-Special Forces. They win the argument. They usually do.

Tuesday, 2 July. At a team meeting, Andy shows the clip of me hobbling my way around the field after being hit by Slipper.

'That's what keeping your line in D means,' he says. 'Eight centimetre tear in his hammy, and still he's in there.'

'I'm not quite sure how you managed that,' Prav whispers to me.

If I wasn't captain I might have gone home, but we're near enough the end of the tour and I want to help in any small way I can. I do my best to be around for the boys without getting in their way. 'We'll win it in even better fashion now,' I tell them. 'What's a week more when this'll last for the rest of our lives?'

I'm saying it to be positive, of course, but there's some truth in it too. As a player, of course you want to close things out as quickly as possible. But you also know that the spectators want nothing more than to have a decider, a shoot-out, and to a degree so do you. To play in a match that will settle everything is such a thrill. If the series is over after two games, whichever side of it you're on, your mind turns to the plane home, even though you've still got one more Test to play. You can't play a Test properly if you're thinking about other things. So a decider keeps the boys keen, and sharp, and honest.

I walk round Sydney in sunglasses and a cap. A decent disguise, I reckon.

'Hello, Sam,' say about a million people.

Turns out my nose really is that big.

Wednesday, 3 July. Gats announces the team. Pence, Tommy, Foxy, Jamie, George, Johnny, Phillsy, Corbs, Hibbs, Bomb, Alun Wyn, Geoff, Lyds, Sean, Toby. Subs: Tom, Mako, Dan, Richie, Tips, Conor, Faz and Manu.

Because people are listening out for their own names, and because even when you know you're not playing you're paying attention to who has been selected rather than who hasn't, it's a moment or two before I realise something.

Drico's been dropped.

Not just from the starting XV, but from the 23 altogether. I wonder whether it's the first time he's ever been dropped from any team. If not, then it must be close. The man's a legend of world rugby.

Foxy's played so well in the first two Tests, and out of position at 12 rather than 13 to boot, that he's made himself pretty much undroppable. Now Jamie's back from his hamstring injury, and he was in great form before that, plus Gats wants his physical presence in the midfield. It's the same reason he's gone for Hibbs at 2 ahead of Tom: Hibbs is the most physical hooker we have, and Gats wants us to impose ourselves wherever we can. Beat them up first, then beat them out wide.

The sentimental thing for Gats to do, of course, would be to put Drico on the bench. But Gats doesn't do sentimental, and in any case Manu can cover 12 and 13 so as a bench option he's more versatile. No one in the camp thinks it's too much of a big deal. We console Drico, of course, and tell him 'hard lines', but people get dropped all the time, no matter who they are.

Back home, it's a different matter entirely. To judge from the reactions, you'd have thought that Gats has done whatever the rugby equivalent of pissing on the Alamo is. Keith Wood calls it a 'terrible mistake'. Willie John McBride says that Australia 'must be laughing all the way' and that the Australian media have convinced Gats to make the decision. David Campese inevitably pops up to say that Gats has 'just handed the series to Australia'. If dropping Drico is the answer, one reporter writes, what on earth is the question?

Gats isn't bothered, or at least he doesn't seem to be. He knows better than anyone that this game is about more than just one player. 'It's only hard because you're making the decision using your head and not your heart,' he says. 'I have to put hand on my heart and say it's the right rugby decision. I would hate to think we had made calls to avoid criticism or for reasons of public popularity.'

And Drico, being a man of substance, reacts just as you'd expect him to. 'Having seen others react in the past to being dropped has given me an insight into how to respond and behave properly. I've seen guys who are dead men walking on tours when they've not been selected and you cannot be that person. The tour is not about you. For you, the decision is huge. For everyone else, you are just one component of it. You deal with your own disappointment in your own way, behind closed doors, but publicly you have to realise that the bigger picture is not your selection, it is about winning the series.

'It is about doing the right thing for everyone, setting the tone around the lads, doing what needs to be done at training, trying to be positive when you have a big inner disappointment. Credit to squad players who have had to do this sort of thing before me, put on the defence bib at training and really mean it out there. It's not easy, keeping your standards up at training. I said all along that it's the contributions of everyone that will make or break the tour. That was true and remains true. Suddenly I am that person. You can't say things one week and then behave differently. You have to suck it up. I hope I'm doing my bit.'

He is. We all are.

Saturday, 6 July. 'It's taken too much out of them to win the second Test,' Gats says. 'They won't peak twice again.'

Andy Farrell surveys the room with steel in his gaze. 'We are taking them boys to the hurt arena.'

In the bus on the way to the ground, I put my headphones on, just as if I were playing. It's the only time in my whole career that I feel this way. Normally when you're not playing you manage to keep some distance. But I'm so involved in this, so desperate for it to end on a high, that I'm every bit as nervous as if I were playing.

Alun Wyn is captain today. He gathers the boys round in the changing-room. 'No separation in defence, no separation in attack. Keep moving. Don't be lazy. Don't give up. And that's not on the 60 or 65, it's from the f***ing first minute to the 80-plus. You don't give up. On a kick-chase. On a jackal. On filling in. You don't give up on anything. For 80 minutes.

'The biggest mark of respect you can have is to be pulled off, blowing out your arse, with nothing left to give. Do not give up on anything. There's a tomorrow with this jersey and one without. We've got 80 minutes to decide which one we want.'

They come out and down the tunnel. I'm screaming at them as they come past. No matter how much I hate match day when I'm playing, I hate it much more when I'm not. It's funny:

I think I'd do anything to get out of it when I do play, but I'd do anything to get back into it when I don't.

The boys come out of the blocks at a rate of knots. Corbs scores from a forwards' drive inside two minutes, and he's so pumped up that he barely notices the congratulations. Two minutes later, Hibbs and George Smith clash heads. Hibbs's blond, Thor-like mane flies everywhere, but he must have a bonce of granite. Smith goes off for a head-injury assessment (HIA) while Hibbs carries on.

Pence keeps the scoreboard ticking over: 10–0, 10–3, 13–3, 16–3, all inside the first quarter of an hour. We're running at more than a point a minute. It's 19–3, when Ben Alexander is sin-binned for persistent infringement at the scrum. Our front row are taking theirs to the cleaners.

Just when we think it might be getting easy, Australia come back. Beale makes a break and it takes two men to bring him down. Then Jesse Mogg comes flying through the middle, and only a desperate tap tackle from Geoff stops him from scoring. Danger signs.

Australia lay siege to our line, and on the stroke of half-time they score, O'Connor taking a high pass, stepping inside Johnny while Tomane bundles Sean out of the way, and then goes through Phillsy and George.

The score is 19–10 at half-time. The biggest lead of the series. But this isn't over yet.

They get another penalty within moments of the restart: 19–13. Then another: 19–16. We need to staunch this. With half an hour left, we get the shunt on at a scrum, and Pence kicks the penalty: 22–16. A bit of breathing space. Not enough.

Finally, we start to play again. Toby steals the ball off Smith, Johnny chips on, George gathers and feeds Foxy, who takes two men with him into touch. From defence to attack in a heartbeat – one of those moments that turns matches, one of those moments that wins series.

We win the lineout and work the phases. Tommy comes off his wing into midfield. Foxy passes to Pence in heavy traffic. Pence dummies and goes. Johnny on his inside, hands out and screaming for the ball. Pence feeds him and Johnny scores, saluting the fans behind the goal: 29–16 with the conversion.

This is ours now.

Pence fields the ball on halfway, dummies again and sets off up the narrow side. Outside Genia. Inside Tomane. Draws Beale and pops it out to George for the score. In the coaches' box, Andy hammers the table in celebration and Rob punches the air. Four minutes later, Conor runs flat, Jamie Roberts runs straight, four men miss him, and he's in too: 41–16.

The Aussie fans begin to stream out of the ground.

I lift the trophy with Alun Wyn. I know I'm tour captain, and I know I've more than played my part – we haven't lost a match when I've been on the pitch – but it still doesn't feel right. I want to have been there in the trenches with the boys, battered and bruised and muddy and sweating, not togged up in my suit as if I'm just off to a drinks party.

If I hadn't had to come off last week, I'd have been man of the match, we'd have clung on to win, and I'd have lifted the trophy in a proper way. Those 'if's again. That's the third year in a row I haven't finished a climactic match, after the World Cup semi in 2011 and the 2012 Grand Slam.

I'm with Paulie and Drico, also in their suits. The three men who'd been tasked with leading the line in the first Test, and now only a fortnight later here we all are, or rather here we all aren't: a broken arm, a torn hamstring and a selection decision. Cruel game. Narrow margins.

'You can't write your own script,' Drico says. 'Other people write it for you.'

Maybe. But now, with the series won and able to call myself not just a winning Lion but a winning Lions captain, I make a small, silent vow to myself.

Sunday, 7 July. Pence and Phillsy are still in the shirts they swapped with Beale and Genia respectively. They haven't slept, they've drunk their own bodyweight in booze, and the shirts haven't been washed. The smell is indescribable.

We're not due to fly home until Tuesday, and the boys make the most of it. They go out three nights in a row, but after the first two I physically can't manage another one. So Lyds and I order room service and have a quiet night in like an old married couple.

Tuesday, 9 July. 'Are you business class or first class?' the Emirates stewardess asks Phillsy.

He gives it a second before giving her a megawatt smile. 'I'm world class.'

The party breaks up in dribs and drabs. Some of the boys get off in Dubai, some in Dublin, some in London. Then it's just us Welsh lot on a bus, and when we see the Severn Bridge we all start singing 'The Green, Green Grass of Home'.

From being on tour with 80 people to driving home in my car alone. Quite a change. Quite a shock. As I pull up outside my front door, I remember the vow I made to myself on the pitch after the victory in Sydney: that in four years' time I'm going to New Zealand, as skipper, to win the series, and to be on the pitch at the end when it happens.

LEADERSHIP 5: POSITIVITY

A leader has to be positive. That was one of the first things Gats saw in me that made him think I could captain Wales: my positivity, the way I was always optimistic and encouraged other people on the pitch.

But there's no point being positive unless you transmit that positivity to the team. In my early days as skipper, I could gee up the boys on the field when I was in game mode and all revved up, but off the pitch it was a different story. I was too quiet, too reserved, and so many of the good things I was feeling didn't really come across.

It was Gethin who brought this to my attention, in his usual brutally blunt way. But that's what I always liked about Gethin. He didn't say things to be a knob, he said them because he felt them and because he thought it would be for the team's benefit. And, as with his on-field reading of the game, he was almost always right.

On this occasion we were sitting in silence outside a cryotherapy chamber, getting changed before going in for our three minutes at 150 degrees below zero. Suddenly, Gethin said: 'You've got to talk more.'

'How do you mean?'

'In meetings and that. You're our captain. You've got to lead us a bit more.'

From then on, I made a point of expressing my positive attitude as much as I could; not to a ridiculous degree but whenever I thought it would have an effect and make a difference. On messy

Monday in 2013, the first time the Lions boys got together, I said to them: 'If someone asks you, "Do you think you'll win the Test series?", that's a bullshit question. The question should be, "Do you *expect* to win the Test series?" And the answer is yes. So when you walk around the hotel with your proud Lions badge on, or in the gym, or when you wake up first thing in the morning, you expect to beat Australia.'

I hated that question, 'Do you think you can win?' In 74 Tests for Wales and five for the Lions, I never once thought beforehand, *We're not going to win this*, no matter who the opposition were. Obviously I had greater success against Australia and New Zealand for the Lions than I did for Wales – in a Welsh shirt I played those two teams a total of 16 times and lost the lot – but even on each of those 16 occasions I thought we'd win before the match. If someone asked me, 'Are you better than New Zealand?', then I said no, clearly we weren't. 'Can you beat them?' Yes, of course. The two things are very different.

Vince Lombardi, the great American football coach, once said that 'you never win a game unless you beat the guy in front of you. You've got to get your man.' I followed this advice every game I played. I'd look at my opposite number before the start. *I'm genetically better than you*, I'd think. *I'm stronger and quicker and more explosive than you. I've trained harder than you, I've eaten better than you, slept better than you, prepared myself better than you. And I've been doing all this since I was 15 years old. I was training on Christmas Day when you were stuffing your face with turkey and falling asleep in front of the TV. I. Am. Better. Than. You.*

But at an even deeper level, being positive involves a shift in mindset. For a long time – for too long – not just Wales but all northern hemisphere sides had an inferiority complex when it came to southern hemisphere opposition. Sir Clive Woodward was the first person really to challenge this. When his England team beat Australia in the 2003 World Cup Final, that was their 12th consecutive win against the big southern hemisphere three, an unbroken run going back to June 2000. Woodward didn't just think he could beat New Zealand, Australia and South Africa; he *expected* to.

Clearly that England side were special, and it would be pointless to expect every side to believe they had the consistent beating of the All Blacks. But what Woodward had also realised is that as often as not, the All Blacks had won matches before they started. Their history, their aura, their kit, their haka – it all added up to a pretty intimidating package. But they're just as human as we are. Everyone feels pain, and anxiety, and pressure. That black jersey is just a jersey. It's not body armour or a superhero's cape. (In fact, Woodward made a point of referring to them only as 'New Zealand', never as the 'All Blacks'.)

For me, then, being positive involved not just thinking that we would win every time out, but that a one-off win against a historically dominant opposition wasn't especially worthy of celebration. Wales haven't beaten New Zealand since 1953. In that time, we've played them 30 times and lost the lot. If you break that sequence and then celebrate madly, that just shows your sense of inferiority. Beat them twice in a short time, as Ireland did to New Zealand in 2016 and 2018? *Then* you can celebrate.

Being positive is about setting standards, not limits. It takes no more energy to have a bigger goal than a smaller one. Gats loved that kind of attitude. So often I'd walk out of one of his team meetings going, 'Yeah, we *are* going to beat X, Y or Z. We *are* better than them at this, that and the other.'

At the launch of the 2014 Six Nations, he wanted me to hold up three fingers while holding the trophy, to signify that we were going to win it that year to go with the two previous ones, but I bottled it. (As it turns out, we didn't win the tournament that year anyway. In fact, in the entire history of the tournament going back to 1883 when it was just the four home nations, no country has ever won three outright titles in a row.)

Gats wanted his players to be confident, and you couldn't be confident if you were feeling negative. At the Spala training camp before the 2011 World Cup, he began one session by saying, 'Right, I want everyone who reckons they'll be in the starting XV for South Africa [our first game of the tournament] to go over there.'

Since no one wanted to look like a bighead who assumed they had a place locked down, no one moved. Except for one person, of course. Phillsy went straight over without hesitation. We were all laughing at him when we noticed Gats nodding in approval: not at us, but at Phillsy. He loved Phillsy's attitude. 'Be positive and back yourself,' he said. 'If you don't back yourself, why should anyone else back you?'

Of course, being positive doesn't mean glossing over things you might prefer not to address. You have to be honest. But be honest in a way that will help improve things, not make them worse. I mentioned in the 'People' section of leadership that you have to know your team not just as a unit but as individuals, and this applies especially when it comes to positivity. Some people need an arm round them now and then; others respond better to tough love.

When Liam Williams first came into the squad, he had a reputation as a bit of a hothead. He had long hair and wasn't afraid of getting involved in aggro; a bit like JPR Williams, except that JPR was a doctor and Liam was a scaffolder. In a team meeting before the 2014 Six Nations match against Scotland, Gats played a video segment comprised entirely of Liam's fouls, penalties conceded, sin-binning and red cards, mainly while he was playing for the Scarlets.

It went on for a couple of minutes, which was a long time when we were all sitting there uncomfortably, feeling awkward for Liam and thinking, *This is random as hell*. At the end, Gats got up, looked down at him and said, 'If you do that for Wales you're going to let all the boys down. You've got to cut it out of your game.'

It might sound a negative things for Gats to have done, and certain players would have crumbled if they'd been on the end of that, but in this case it was quite the opposite. First, he knew Liam was tough enough to take it. Second, the positive side of Liam's play – his brilliance under the high ball and his running – was built into this. If he hadn't been as talented as he was, Gats wouldn't have bothered to go to all this effort. He'd have just dropped him from the squad. Third, it was a message to all of us that no one could afford to have this stuff in their own game. Fourth, and most of all, it worked. I can hardly remember a yellow card Liam's had since.

In essence, it was Gats's way of saying, 'Mate, I've got your back, but only if you've got mine.' That kind of positive reinforcement, everyone bolstering everyone else, is crucial in a team environment. Early in the second Lions Test against Australia in 2013, Mako Vunipola was having a torrid time with referee Craig Joubert.

'I don't know how many scrum penalties I gave away in that first 10 to 20 minutes,' Mako said. 'The scrums then affected the rest of my game. I became uptight and started doing things I usually don't. Opportunities to pass the ball, I hold the ball. I'm second-guessing what to do. I could feel myself kind of closing off.'

What helped him through was the support of his team-mates, especially his fellow front-row members. 'Tom Youngs was massive that day in giving me the confidence to keep going, to do what I can. Adam Jones kept telling me, "Don't worry, mate, I've got you."' Mako rode out the storm that day, and became a much better and more confident player in the long run.

It's not just the team on the pitch who can do their bit for positivity; it's everyone. The video boys did us a little segment of our greatest hits (literally and metaphorically), which they played just before our 2013 match against England. Keeping journalists onside and getting them to buy into the team's success can really help too. Of course they need to sell papers, and of course they're entitled to criticise when they see things they don't like, but there's a difference between justified, constructive criticism and sarcastic carping from the sidelines.

People in general respond better to positivity than to negativity, to being reinforced rather than undermined. A positive team is more likely to be a confident team; a confident team is more likely to be a successful one. Every team will come under pressure, and being positive about that is the single best way of dealing with it.

There are three common reactions to pressure: fight, flight and freeze. It's the leader's job to ensure that both he and everyone on his team always responds with the first of these rather than either of the latter two.

This is easier said than done. Even – especially – in professional sport, there are plenty of people who don't fancy every challenge. I've heard more than my fair share of creative excuses from boys who wanted to duck a particular game for whatever reason (often the fear of being shown up by their opposite number). One even pulled out the old 'dog ate my passport' line.

And this doesn't necessarily have anything to do with how successful or not the team in question is. One player from the Liverpool football team of the 1980s said that at least half his team-mates couldn't wait for 4.45 on a Saturday. That team won everything going – league titles, FA Cups, European Cups – yet the players still felt the pressure so acutely that they couldn't wait for it to be over, at least for a few days until the next match.

That pressure is relentless. When you're not top dog, you're trying to be top dog. When you are top dog, you're trying to stay there. So how do you ensure that pressure brings out the best in you rather than the worst? How do you ensure that you neither run away (flight) or go through the motions (freeze), but instead meet the challenge with everything you have (fight)?

As with most other aspects of leadership, it starts with your mindset. One of the sportsmen I most admire is Michael Johnson, the great American 200-metre and 400-metre runner. 'Pressure,' he once said, 'is the shadow of great opportunity.' I'm not that big on using inspirational quotes, but this was one that really struck me and stayed with me.

Pressure is the shadow of great opportunity.

People often perceive pressure as a bad thing. But if there's pressure, it's often because something really good can come of it. When people are nervous, they tend to focus on the bad things that might happen. In my case, this could have been any number of things. *We might lose. I might play badly. I might do something that costs my team the match. I might get injured. I might play so badly or get so badly injured that my career's over.*

Instead, I would focus on and chase down the good that could come of this pressure, this opportunity. I would get excited about what could go right rather than worry about what could go wrong. *We're going to win. I'm going to play well. I'm going to be man of the match. We're going to set our names in stone as one of the greatest Lions teams ever.*

Don't be afraid of what you could lose. Be excited about what you could achieve. You've got to be brave, take chances and make things happen. When you get to the real big games, you don't want the occasion to inhibit the players. You still want them to have a go, play with freedom and instinct.

If you see pressure as a threat, you won't perform to your optimum. Seeing pressure as a threat undermines your self-confidence, impairs your judgement and increases the likelihood that you'll try something impulsive and high risk that is much more likely to go wrong than go right – and which may well end up bringing about exactly the kind of negative outcome you feared to start with.

If you see pressure as a challenge, on the other hand, all those things will be reversed. You'll be more confident and your brain will be working at a higher level, making your judgement more rather than less reliable. Rather than rush into things in the *hope* that they'll go well, you'll take a little more time in the *expectation* that they'll go well. This also helps you assess all the available information and make considered decisions.

That's why goalkickers go through their routines before each kick, to make pressure work *for* them rather than *against* them. Jenks, talking about the five penalties he kicked in the titanic second 1997 Lions Test, which won them the series, said: 'The pressure mounted with each kick, but every time I took my mind away from Durban and imagined myself back on my training field in Church Village. Same routine and, thankfully, same result. People always ask about pressure kicks, but that is what goalkickers live for. You don't hope the chance never comes; you pray it does.'

You don't hope the chance never comes; you pray it does.

Business executives often use stress balls for a good reason: squeezing them activates the parts of the brain that control unconscious responses, while suppressing the parts of the brain that govern self-conscious thinking. Clearly I didn't have a stress ball to squeeze in the heat of a Test match (even if some of my French opponents seemed to like using parts of my anatomy for that purpose), but I would try to follow the same principles.

Almost every time I had to make a decision in a match, I'd remind myself I had more time than I thought I did. It could be hard to remember that when the adrenaline was flying, the crowd were roaring and the oppo were chopsing off at you, but all those were irrelevant. The only person whose word I had to take was the ref, and if I was taking too long he'd tell me.

Of course, it's not enough just to turn up on the day and think you can put these kind of things into practice. You have to train for them, just like you train for fitness and skills. In fact, we'd often do our skills sessions immediately after a savage fitness block to get us used to making decisions when we were fatigued and under pressure.

Then we'd make it harder by having coaches and other players shouting at us and trying to distract us when we were, for example, rehearsing lineout calls. If we couldn't get things right under those conditions, we weren't going to be able to do so with 78 minutes gone in a Test and 60,000 fans yelling their heads off.

Clive Woodward called it T-CUP – Thinking Clearly Under Pressure – and the England team that won the World Cup in 2003 practised that over and over again. Indeed, it was T-CUP that won them that trophy. If you examine the move that led to Jonny Wilkinson's decisive drop goal – a score that came after 99 minutes of one of the most intense Test matches imaginable, and therefore at a time when every man on the pitch must have been exhausted – you can see several examples of T-CUP in quick succession:

- Steve Thompson throws long to the back of the lineout, knowing that Australia will bank on him making what they think is a risky call and therefore won't be as likely to steal the ball off the jumper Lewis Moody.
- From a ruck, Matt Dawson knows both that the Aussie players will be flat on the offside line to try to charge down a drop-kick, and that England are still too far out for Wilkinson to play the percentages and waste what might be their last chance. So Dawson shows and goes, making 10 metres and putting Wilkinson within range.
- Martin Johnson, the skipper, calls for the ball off this ruck. He's not doing this to make yards or change the play. He's doing it because Neil Back's at scrum-half while Dawson's still on the ground, and because England need Dawson – their best passer – in place for the drop goal attempt. Back passes short to Johnson, who takes the contact and allows Dawson to get back in position.
- Dawson goes to pass. The Aussie defenders start to charge, but when they see that the ball's still in the ruck, they have to go back behind the offside line – and it's at that moment, when they're back on their heels and Dawson's bought Wilkinson an extra half-second, that the scrum-half fires the pass out to Wilkinson.
- Wilkinson hasn't got the angle to hit the kick with his favoured left foot and be sure of it going over. So he takes it

onto his right foot and hits it with that one. It's not the prettiest kick in the world. But if you're an English fan, it's just about the best thing you've ever seen on a rugby pitch.

Of course, there was more to all this than just thinking clearly under pressure. England needed the fitness, skill and teamwork to back it up. But when you add it all together, you see that pressure didn't cow them; it inspired them, all the way to the greatest prize in this sport.

6

TWICKENHAM

51.4559°N, 0.3415°W

**Saturday, 26 September 2015. England v Wales,
World Cup Pool A match**

*Three minutes left. Mike Brown takes it up into contact. I'm
on him like a flash. This is mine, sunshine. This is my
turnover.*

Jérôme Garcès blows. 'Red 7, not releasing.'

*I can't believe my ears. That was a legitimate jackal all day
long.*

Don't argue. The referee's word is law.

*George Ford sets his body away from the posts. They're not
going for three points and the draw; they're going for the
corner and the try, and that is an insult to every single player
in a red jersey on this pitch. We don't think a draw's good
enough, that's what England are saying. We don't think you've
got it in you to hold us out.*

Right. Bring it on. Bring it on.

*Ford drills it into touch on our five-metre line. We set
ourselves for the lineout while the England forwards take their*

time, walking slowly upfield, knowing this is their big chance, and wanting, needing, to get it right.

*I march up and down our line like a sergeant major at Rorke's Drift. 'No way they get this! Stand your ground. Stand your ground! No f***** comes through here.'*

Saturday, 28 September. Tottenham v Chelsea, White Hart Lane. We're invited to watch the match from one of the hospitality boxes. A club official asks me if I'll come down at half-time to be introduced to the crowd. No way, I say. He says they'd really like to, and after the Lions victory in Australia I'm sure to get a good reception. I'm not so sure – the vast majority of Spurs supporters surely couldn't give a toss about rugby – but eventually I agree.

They take me down to the pitch side just before the break, so I get to see the players coming in at half-time: chatting, laughing, having a go at each other, just like I'm used to. Then I'm brought out onto the pitch and they announce my name. I've got my tail between my legs, convinced that no one's going to know who the hell I am and I'm going to be greeted with an embarrassing silence.

There's a huge cheer, followed by a prolonged round of applause. I can't believe it. This is the club I've supported for the best part of 20 years, and here they are welcoming me as though I was playing for them. It's one of the highlights of my career, it really is.

They interview me on the pitch.

'Tell us about your dogs, Sam.'

'I'm such a fan that all my dogs have been named after Spurs players. I've had Glenn after Glenn Hoddle, Ted and Gus after Teddy Sheringham and Gus Poyet, Dawson after Michael Dawson, Alfie after Alfie Conn, the first player my dad ever saw score, and now we've got Ledley.' Ledley King retired last year, plagued by a knee injury so bad that he couldn't even train; he'd just turn up every Saturday and still play everyone else off the park.

'Doesn't your fiancée get a say in all this?'

'Ha! I can't tell you the number of names she came up with this time. But I just said it has to be Ledley. He's my all-time hero.'

'Why do you like him so much?'

'He was just so classy, on the ball and off it. I can't remember him making a mistake. He never put a foot wrong. He played in my old position, central defence, and like me he had more than his share of injuries. And I love the fact he was a one-club man. I've only ever played my professional club rugby for Cardiff Blues, and I hope I only ever will. I'm very proud to be Cardiff.'

'That's great, Sam. Thank you very much.'

I turn to go back up to the box – and standing there in front of me, holding a Tottenham shirt with **WARBURTON 7** on the back, is Ledley King himself.

I'm dumbstruck and starstruck. I'm so nervous that my leg's shaking. I know, I know. I'm a grown man. I'm Lions captain. But I have my heroes just like everyone else, and Ledley King is mine. I want to ask if we can have a photo together, but I can't get the words out. Luckily Ledley realises that's what I want, and so we pose together for a snap.

I go back up to the box grinning like a loon. Dad's filmed it all on his phone. I ask to see the footage. While all the Spurs fans are applauding, I see the Chelsea fans are giving me the wanker sign. Some things never change.

I told the Spurs interviewer that I wanted to be a one-club man until the end of my career, and I mean it, but increasingly it seems as though things on that front might be out of my control.

It's no secret that the WRU has been at loggerheads with the four regional teams (the Blues, the Dragons, the Scarlets and the Ospreys) for some time now. I try to keep out of the politics as much as possible – there's little I can do to influence things even if I wanted to, and I know it would be a huge distraction to my training and game preparation if I did get involved – but it's hard to avoid all of it when you know it may have direct implications for your career.

To cut a (very) long story short, players' contracts are with their regions, not the WRU. When those contracts are up, the best players find themselves offered more money – sometimes much more – by clubs in England and France. Careers are short, and players have every right to maximise their earning potential. But the trickle overseas has now become a flood. George has gone to Northampton; Phillsy, Jamie and Lyds to Racing Métro; Hooky to Perpignan; and Foxy to Clermont Auvergne.

The WRU is proposing to stop this by centrally contracting the elite players themselves and loaning them back to the regions at no cost. Sounds like a great deal for the regions, right? Not as far as they're concerned. They fear that if the

WRU control elite players' contracts they'll also control where and when those players can play, with the needs of the national team always taking precedence over those of the regions. No region wants to pick an international player for an important Heineken Cup match, say, only to be told they can't have him.

From a player's point of view, this is manna from heaven. At the moment we're pieces of meat, more or less. Sure, club coaches care about player welfare, but they care more about winning games. In a 50–50 call, you're always going to be under pressure to play. And players do themselves no favours by acting all alpha and playing through injury when they shouldn't. Central contracts would take care of all this. Central contracts would mean proper rest.

The WRU will want a player for maybe a dozen matches a season, with more in World Cup years. A club will want that same player for two or three times that many games. 'Rest' means different things to club than it does to country. Add to this a lack of trust and a whole host of tensions between the various sides – Blues chairman Peter Thomas saying the WRU 'couldn't run a corner shop', the regions saying they don't get enough funding from the WRU and looking at signing some kind of deal with England's Aviva Premiership – and you can see why Welsh rugby's garden is a lot more thorns than roses.

I want to continue to play for the Blues if at all possible. I'm Wales captain, a role I take very seriously, and I think it's really important that a country's captain should play his rugby in that country. But like everyone else I've got my own career to consider, and there's at least one French club that's coming in hard for me. The richest of them all, with the largest collection of famous players on its books, the Real Madrid of rugby: Toulon.

Even the mention of Toulon makes people think it's about the money. It's not. It never has been for me, in any walk of life. If I'd been that motivated by money I'd have gone to an English club and earned three times as much as I do for the Blues. I'm not that materialistic – my idea of extravagance is putting an extra bedroom into our semi-detached house – and I know I'll be able to earn money after my playing career's over.

But it *is* about success, as it should be for any rugby player who takes the game seriously. Toulon are Heineken Cup champions. The nearest I've got to club success with Cardiff has been as a sub in the 2010 Amlin Challenge Cup victory, when we overcame massive odds to beat – ironically – Toulon in the final. The prospect of winning serious silverware, and continuing to improve my game by playing week in, week out with Toulon's squad, is pretty enticing.

I go over to Toulon with Derwyn to have a look. Jonny Wilkinson comes to have a chat. He's loving it here, and it shows: he looks tanned, happy and relaxed, much more so than he usually did in an England shirt. The weather's great, the old town is charming, and everyone is beautifully dressed and rocking the Vincent Clerc-style sexy French accents.

What's not to love?

Well, two things. One, I'd be expected to play for Toulon like I do for Wales, and probably about 30 times a season to boot. I don't know if my body's up to it. The Blues are used to the way I play for them, and they're very understanding and accepting of it, but I don't know whether Toulon would be so forgiving, especially with the money they'd be forking out.

Second, I'm a homeboy. The Mediterranean lifestyle looks idyllic, but at home in Rhiwbina I have everything I need:

my entire family living within half a mile of each other, the woods where I can walk the dog and look out over Cardiff Bay, the Juboraj for a Friday-night curry. I'd miss all that. I'd really miss it.

I don't say no to Toulon. I'd still prefer to stay in Wales. But if the WRU and the regions can't sort themselves out, and I feel that staying put will be detrimental to my career, I'll be off.

Saturday, 30 November. Once again we play Australia. Once again it's a great match, full of tension and incidents. Once again it's close: we're within four points of them for the last 12 minutes.

And once again we lose.

I suffer another shoulder stinger. I'm out until the start of the Six Nations, two months away. Injury #12.

The *Lions Raw* DVD comes out: the official documentary of the Lions' Australia tour, with lots of behind-the-scenes footage.

Rach's parents, who from next summer will be my in-laws, are shocked to see me ranting and raving before the first Test, shouting at the boys in the changing-room. 'If they're into you, you f***ing pile 'em. Every single f***ing bastard collision. Get up off the floor, work f***ing hard for your team-mates.'

'That's not what Sam's like,' Rach's mum says.

Ben laughs. 'That's *exactly* what Sam's like.'

Friday, 24 January 2014. Toulon have asked me to make a decision by 10 pm. Derwyn's passed that deadline on to the WRU, who are still trying to work out the mechanics of central contracts, and told them that if we don't have an offer from them by that time then I'm signing for Toulon.

I want to stay in Wales. I want to sign a central contract – it would be the first central contract ever awarded in Wales, and I guess it would be fitting for the national captain to sign it – and I don't want the WRU to suffer the negative publicity that my departure would bring them.

But if they can't offer me anything, I can't hang around waiting forever.

Derwyn and I are at a dinner. Lots of small talk and pressing the flesh, but all the time we're waiting for our phones to vibrate in our pockets with an email from the WRU's chief executive Roger Lewis.

Eight o'clock comes and goes.

Eight-thirty.

Nine.

Now and then I catch Derwyn's eye and raise my eyebrows: *You got anything?* And each time he shakes his head.

At nine-thirty our phones buzz and we grab them simultaneously.

Dear Sam. We are delighted to be able to offer you a central contract with the WRU ...

Derwyn and I high-five each other. It would have been easy for him, since he takes a percentage of my deals, to have pushed me towards Toulon and just gone for the big bucks. But he didn't, and he never has. I remember the first time we met, back when I was in the Blues academy, and we talked about managing my career long-term, not just chasing the newest and shiniest thing on offer.

He's been as good as his word, every step of the way. He laid out the advantages and disadvantages of going to Toulon, set up the trip there and the meetings so I could see the place for myself, but he's always made it very clear that the final decision must be mine and mine alone. He's been there for all the shit times as well as all the good ones. I'm very lucky to have him, not just as an agent but as a mate too.

And if I told him that, he'd roll his eyes, tut, and go, 'Don't be a soft cock.'

Saturday, 25 January. I sign the contract with Roger in front of reporters and photographers. The final details of the WRU's agreement with the Blues haven't quite been hammered out – the intention is that the WRU and the Blues split my wage bill 60/40 – but Roger assures us that it'll all go through fine.

I take Ledley for a walk, and I can hardly go ten yards without someone congratulating me or beeping their car horn as they drive past. My Twitter feed is full of positive comments too, though perhaps inevitably there are a couple of people saying that Ospreys players would never have done this, calling me a traitor to the Blues, that kind of thing. It doesn't bother me. Anyone who knows me knows how much I love the Blues.

Financially, my decision has cost me, as I would have earned double if I'd left for Toulon.

Of course, I'd have earned international appearance fees and sponsorship endorsements either way, so overall I'd have been well remunerated whether I'd gone to France or stayed in

Wales, but if it was purely about the cash I'd have been off to Toulon. I've never made a single decision based on money, and I'm not going to start now.

Saturday, 1 February. A little short of match fitness after my injury, I'm on the bench against Italy at the Millennium. With 16 minutes to go, I come on for Lyds.

'On for Wales, number 20, Sam Warburton,' says the announcer.

The crowd roar louder than I've ever heard them before. If I doubted for one minute that I did the right thing in turning down Toulon, here's the proof. They so appreciate that I've chosen to stay in Wales, and this is their way of showing that.

I have tears in my eyes as I run across the pitch to the lineout.

Saturday, 15 March. Last minute of the match against Scotland. We've absolutely annihilated them – 51–3, seven tries – but I'm so determined to keep going right until the end, Terminator-style, that I hit a ruck with only a few seconds left as hard as I'd hit one with only a few seconds gone.

Too hard, as it turns out. There's a sudden spike of agony in my shoulder, and the physios come racing on. I've dislocated my shoulder and torn my labrum.

Injury #13. Three months out, which means no summer tour of South Africa. The damage is so bad that I won't be able to lift jumpers in the lineout for another two years.

* * *

It's funny how my attitude to injuries has changed. At the start of my career they seemed like the end of the world, as though even the slightest knock would undo all the years of training and playing. Now, a dozen injuries in, I'm much more sanguine about it all.

For a start, injury means rest, not just physically but mentally too. The mental side of building yourself towards a peak every Saturday, coming crashing down after a match and then gradually building again during the week is much harder than people think.

There's always something you can do while you're injured. You can get yourself fit in other ways, boosting parts of the body that aren't affected by your injury. This bit has never been hard for me; I love training so much that I used to do my own pre-preseason, if that makes sense.

But no matter who you are, rehab is hard. You're out of the team environment, and you feel that absence acutely. It's not just that you're not there; it's that someone else is there in your place, wearing your shirt, making your tackles, hitting your rucks, winning your turnovers, and the longer you're out the more chance they have of staking a permanent claim to your spot.

Then again, you know that it happens to everyone sooner or later, and more than once. What you're going through now, someone else will be going through themselves soon enough. I remember seeing an interview with Drico back when I was 15 or so in which he said he'd never played 100 per cent fit. *Bollocks*, I thought at the time. *That must be bollocks. He's just saying that to make himself look hard.*

Now I realise how true it is. The 2011 Six Nations was the nearest I've got to taking the field without any problems whatsoever. Other than that, there's always something. I try not to take painkillers in training – pain is the body's way of telling you something's wrong, and when your body is your career then you need to listen – but sometimes in matches you have no choice if you want to get through them.

And here's what you don't see when you see me running around the pitch smashing into rucks like a mad thing. You don't see me having to crawl up the stairs on all fours after a game, as I simply can't walk up them. You don't see the way I walk across the landing to the bathroom when I've just woken up, all stiff and gingerly as though I'm treading barefoot on broken glass. You don't see the headaches that can last for days. And you don't see that I have to sleep on my back every night; I can't sleep on my shoulders because they're too sore.

I could sleep on my front, I guess, but my nose gets in the way.

Sunday, 22 June. I'm at home, but over in Singapore some of the Blues boys are playing in the first ever World Cup Tens tournament. Owen Williams is one of them. He's a young lad, 22 years of age, but he's already played for Wales four times at outside centre, and he's an absolute specimen: George North apart, probably the single best athlete I've ever played with.

The Blues are playing the Asia-Pacific Dragons for third place, a nothing match, and Owen's hit in a nothing tackle. But he falls awkwardly, and when he hits the ground it's as though he's a hand puppet with the strings let go. His limbs just drop.

It's not a bad injury. It's a catastrophic one. He's damaged his cervical vertebrae and spinal cord. He's left paraplegic, with no feeling in his legs and torso and only a fraction of what he once had in his arms. It's a week before he can even be flown home, where he'll spend the best part of a year in hospital.

For everyone at the Blues, it's the most horrendous thing. We all know that there but for the grace of God go any of us; a freak accident, a one-in-a-billion chance, an apparently innocuous moment that changes everything forever. You can take all the safety precautions you like, and one random act of chance makes them irrelevant.

I'm not especially close to Owen, but what's happened to him really affects me. It's there in the back of my mind the whole time. Practising on the scrum machine, doing tackling drills; like all the boys I leap up from those twice as fast as I did before, just in case.

At three in the morning, when the darkness is there in every way, done for life, thinking, *this is forever* … I can't even bring myself to go there. The poor, poor lad.

Saturday, 5 July. Rach and I get married – a church service in Newport followed by a reception at the Celtic Manor resort, which hosted the Ryder Cup four years ago.

Rach looks absolutely beautiful. It's a cliché, but like all clichés it's one because it's true: it's the happiest day of my life. All the people I love are here, and everyone's laughing and drinking and having a great time. We keep the day pretty much totally private – I tweet a handful of pictures, no more – and a couple of papers run some wedding photos of other Welsh rugby players by way of comparison.

I definitely couldn't pull off the white suit look the way Andy Powell does, and Gareth Edwards has sideburns I can only dream of. Best of all, though, was Rupert Moon, whose wedding was attended by Lance Corporal William Windsor, the official goat of the Royal Welsh!

Saturday, 22 November. Owen comes to watch us play the All Blacks at the Millennium. The crowd stand and applaud him as one. His resilience and determination are an inspiration to everyone, players and fans alike.

George North is feeling down after the match, and it's not just because we've lost again.

'I've had another concussion,' he says to Lyds and me. 'I got hit in the head, and for half a second I didn't know where I was or which way I was supposed to be playing.'

Lyds and I look at each other and burst out laughing.

'Mate,' Lyds says, 'that happens to us literally every game.'

It does, too. I've lost count of the number of times I've taken a knock to the head, got up and not been sure which way I'm playing. Normally I just look to see what the guys wearing the same coloured jerseys as me are doing, and work it out from there. If there's a lineout straight after the knock, I'll tell the caller not to send any to the back as I can't remember the call signs for a minute or two. If play's still going through the phases, I just hit the next ruck or take up my position in the defensive line, as those are by now more muscle memory and instinct than actual mental recall.

Never go off unless you're injured.

And a blow to the head, unless you're actually unconscious, doesn't count.

In years to come, I'll look back and think how frightening it was that we knew so little. We appreciate how serious things like spinal injuries are, of course, but not head knocks. That's one of the biggest differences I've seen from the start of my career to the end of it, the way in which head injuries are dealt with. The *Mail on Sunday* has started running a campaign to highlight the dangers of concussion, and slowly the message is filtering through to the game and the players.

Saturday, 29 November. Three minutes left. We're leading South Africa 12–6. They've got a scrum on our five-metre line.

We set ourselves. We have to hold out. These are the times when we've lost so often to the southern hemisphere sides: right at the end, in the clutch, when we've done all the hard work but don't quite have the nous, the bottle, the bloody-mindedness, call it what you like, to finish the job off.

We get the wheel on, disrupt them. Toby comes away with the ball. We clear our lines. All that matters now is that we play the rest of the game in their half. They can have the ball all they like, as long as we have the territory.

Willie le Roux has it. He's one of the most dangerous broken-field runners in world rugby. Their half or ours, he can conjure something from nothing.

He knocks on.

One minute left. We have possession. We spill it. *Not again. Please, not again.* Wales have lost their last 16 games to South Africa. Wales haven't beaten South Africa this century, this millennium even. Wales have suffered 22 successive defeats against New Zealand, South Africa and Australia.

The Boks run it from deep. We're frantically covering. They work it down the left-hand side. Fast passes. Flat passes. Too flat, that last one, surely?

One whistle for the forward pass, and then two for full-time. *We've won.* It takes a moment to sink in. *We've actually bloody won.*

It's been intense and ferocious, but it hasn't been a great game: six penalties, no tries. I don't care. It's my first victory against one of the big three in 16 attempts, and that alone makes it one of the best days of my career, even though I've suffered another shoulder stinger. Injury #14.

Saturday, 10 January 2015. Cardiff Blues v Leinster, Pro 12. Eleven minutes gone. Leinster take it off the top of a lineout and send Ben Te'o hammering up the middle. He's wearing a cast on his forearm, and as I go to tackle him he leads with that arm and clobbers me in the face. I'm knocked backwards, and as I get up I see that Josh Navidi's made the tackle from behind, so I go in to jackal.

I can't see a thing.

There's blood running down inside my eye socket. I can't even blink, as my eyelid's split. The ref looks at me and his face goes white. *Jeez, it must look bad.* And that makes me panic a bit. If there are two things I'm scared of, it's injuries to my teeth and my eyes. The rest of it I take as an occupational hazard, but those two really freak me out.

The medics take me off. One of them washes my eye in sterile solution and then stitches the cut. Because I can't close my eye, I've no choice but to watch the needle all the way.

'Don't worry,' he says, as though reading my mind. 'I do this for a living.'

I do what I do for a living too, I think, *but there have to be easier ways than this.*

I ask for a tissue. The moment I blow my nose, there's another sharp fork of pain and my eye swells up like a balloon.

'Ah,' says the medic. 'That's red flag for a fracture.'

Injury #15.

I make a mental note. Ben Te'o: I won't forget this.

Saturday, 21 March. Last day of the Six Nations, and three teams are still in the mix for the championship: England, Ireland and us. We each have three wins out of four.

The matches are staggered, which makes sense from the TV point of view but is also unfair: the team that goes last will know exactly what it has to do to win the championship. Unfortunately, we're first up at lunchtime in Rome. We stick a hatful of points on Italy, beating them 60–21.

Ireland are next, knowing they have to beat Scotland by 20 points at Murrayfield to overhaul us on points difference. At half-time they're right on track, leading 20–10, but any hope we have that Scotland might be able to keep the gap down vanishes ten minutes later when Johnny Sexton converts a Jared Payne try to put Ireland 30–10 up. They end up winning 40–10, and that's our chance gone.

England now need to beat France by 26 points to finish ahead of Ireland, and they so nearly do it in an insane match at Twickenham. It ends 55–35, with England scoring seven tries and France five, and at times it's almost like watching a sevens match.

For the fans, it's been brilliant – the most exciting last day in Six Nations history for many a year. But I can't help feeling that the schedule robbed us of our chance. By winning so big so early, we forced Ireland and England to go out and play. If we'd played last, or even if we'd all played simultaneously, they'd have been much more conservative: we were only a point up on Italy at half-time. I know there's no way round this, and the best way to avoid being in situations like this is simply to win all your matches and not need to worry about results elsewhere.

In any case, we've got bigger fish to fry.

The World Cup's just around the corner, and I honestly feel we can do even better than we did last time round. We're more experienced, we're more battle-hardened, we've got a great nucleus of boys who've played together for the past few years and know each other's games inside out.

The Group of Death looks even harder now than it did back when the draw was made in 2012. Australia, England and us are now ranked second, third and fourth in the world now. Three potential semi-finalists in one group, with only two to go through. And my determination is the same now as it was the day the draw was made: we're going to be one of those two, whatever it takes.

Whatever it takes, part one. Wales training camp at altitude in the Swiss resort of Fiesch. Fast feet on a box while holding a water bag whose constantly shifting weight keeps unbalancing me and making me use my core. I go over on my ankle. The press are there, filming and interviewing us. I can't let them know that I'm hurt.

The next drill is a 30-metre run. I whisper to the physios that I'll do this, and then can they give me some different exercises from the others so as not to alert the reporters? The run's agony, but I just about make it through, and then the physios tell me to lie on my back and do some leg exercises that don't involve any weight bearing.

When the press have gone, the physios take a proper look. My ankle's black and blue. Grade 2+ ligament tear. Injury #16.

And that's not even the worst thing about the camp. We sleep much higher than we train, and we have to take a cable car between the two. It runs high above the treeline of dark green conifers, and since I'm terrified of heights I spend most of each trip sprawled out on the floor like a tarantula.

The boys are sympathetic, of course. In roughly the same way that Hannibal Lecter's sympathetic.

Whatever it takes, part two. Wales training camp, Doha, high summer. 'Hot' doesn't even begin to describe it. It's murderous, a living thing, the kind of heat that reaches out and smacks you in the face the second you go outside. It's mid-forties and 95 per cent humidity to boot: one giant steam room, all day long.

You know you're in for a tough training session when you see an ambulance and paramedics waiting by the side of the pitch before you even begin.

The coaches flog us mercilessly. Training in these conditions will help us produce more red blood cells, which will in turn increase our oxygen-carrying capacity and allow us to keep going for longer in matches, but just as importantly they want to see whether we have the mental toughness to cope with such conditions.

Everyone suffers. Tomas Francis needs to be given oxygen and covered with soaking wet towels to bring his temperature down. The session ends with a drill where we have to run to halfway and back in 20 seconds, followed by 20 seconds rest, repeated five times.

Jamie can't do it. They bring his cones back by five metres, then five metres more, and so on until he's jogging 10 metres back and forth at a snail's pace. But he never stops. He never gives up. That's what they're looking for. Just as in Spala four years ago, these are the experiences that we'll draw on in the measureless depths of a hard match. I've never seen anyone with an oxygen mask on at half-time in the Millennium, put it that way.

Play hard. Train harder.

Whatever it takes, part three. Full-contact training back at the Arms Park. Jake Ball comes flying into a ruck and smacks me. He's one of our very best cleanout players, and he gets me right on the shoulder where I've been done so often before. That evening, sharing with Lyds, I can't lift my arm up to put a T-shirt on.

I go down to see the physios. They're in with the coaches, and I don't want the coaches to know just yet. I ask Prav if I can have a word. He gives me a quick assessment. Another month out, he says. Injury #17.

* * *

Morale is high as the tournament gets nearer. Andre, our chef, sets up bushtucker trials, offering a choice of delicacies like pig's nose or a pint of mashed-up ear against the forfeit of more training. *I'm a Welsh Rugby Player, Get Me Out of Here!*

Our conditioning coach Paul Stridgeon – everyone calls him Bobby after Adam Sandler's character in *The Waterboy* – awards the Bobby Cup every week to someone who's done something good, on or off the pitch. Thierry Henry's training at the Vale with the Welsh football team, so Bobby asks him if he'll do a short video announcing the winner of this week's Bobby Cup.

Thierry's clearly a good lad, despite being a Gunner, as he says sure, he'd be delighted. We're all in a team meeting when he comes on the screen. 'Allo, boys,' he says, sounding even more French than Vincent Clerc. 'Ze winner of ze Bobby Cup ees ...' big 10-second pause ... 'Nicky Smith!' Then he looks straight into the camera, winks and goes 'va-va-voom.'

Nicky's the source of general amusement anyway. Jamie clocked that Nicky's terrible at spelling, so at each team meeting he gets Nicky to stand up while Jamie reads out a word for him to spell. The word appears on the screen behind Nicky, so we can see it but he can't.

'When you finally get one right,' we tell him, 'you've got to get Jamie back.'

Eventually Nicky does get one right, to huge applause.

'Right,' he tells Jamie. 'You've been rinsing me long enough. Your turn.'

Up comes Jamie. He turns to face us. Rhys Webb's already primed the video boys. They put up a picture of Jamie taken from above in a match. His hair's thinning, which is even more obvious when his head's wet and sweaty. We all piss ourselves laughing.

'Since you're a doctor,' Nicky says, 'I'm going to give you a medical term.'

'Bring it on,' Jamie says.

The word comes up on the screen as Nicky reads it out. 'Jamie, can you spell "hair transplant"?'

Everyone's creasing themselves, Jamie included. He takes it really well, and of course spells it perfectly.

These are the things that get you through hard training camps: suffer with your team-mates on the pitch, and laugh with them off it.

Wednesday, 23 September. We arrive at Oatlands Park in Surrey, where we'll be based until we play England on Saturday. I'm sharing with Lyds, as usual.

'Is it me, or is this place a bit creepy?' I say as we're unpacking.

'It's not you,' Lyds replies. 'It's haunted.'

Lyds is quite receptive to this kind of stuff. He's experienced paranormal activity in the old bit of his family's farmhouse in mid-Wales.

'You're winding me up,' I say.

'Google it and find out.'

So I do. And guess what? Turns out that Oatlands Park is one of the five most haunted hotels in the south of England. Great.

I read all the stories I can find. The really haunted room, apparently, is the one right next to ours, where one of the physios is sleeping, but there's still a weird energy in our room that I don't like.

Later that night, I'm dropping off to sleep when …

… bang!

I'm sitting up in a flash, shitting myself. Lyds likes to sleep with the curtains open, so there's a bit of natural light coming in, enough for me to see him half upright with his neck fully extended, as though he's looking at something.

I'm too scared to move a muscle or say a word.

Gradually Lyds lies back down, and so do I. I lie awake for hours, and it's only around three in the morning that I drift into an uneasy sleep.

Bang! Bang! Bang!

I'm out of bed again like a shot. It's 6 am. The noises are coming from the door. I go over and open it.

It's the drugs testers.

When they've taken our samples, I look for my phone. It's nowhere to be seen. I don't even dare joke that the ghost took it.

Eventually I find it on the floor, next to the skirting board. That bang I heard last night must have been the phone falling off the table onto the floor. But the phone was in the middle of the table and it wasn't on vibrate, so how did it fall?

Thursday, 24 September. It's 10.30 pm. I'm drifting off to sleep again when suddenly Lyds throws his sheets off and sits bolt upright, staring in front of him. I can't see anything.

'Lyds?' I say.

He doesn't answer.

'Lyds,' I say again. 'Lyds.' Louder. 'Lyds, you're freaking me out.'

He's frozen for about 20 seconds, and then he slowly turns his head and looks at me.

'There's a man sitting on the end of my bed looking at me.'

I still can't see anyone or anything. There's no one in the room apart from us.

'Mate,' I say, trying to keep my voice steady, 'are you asleep? Maybe you're sleep-talking or something.'

'I'm wide awake.'

'I don't see a thing.'

'There's a man sitting on my bed ...'

'I saw a Derren Brown thing about this once ...'

'... wearing old-fashioned gear ...'

'... about your brain being really active before sleep, and you probably saw a picture in the hotel earlier ...'

'... and he's looking at me.' Pause. 'He's gone.'

Friday, 25 September. We go down to breakfast. The first thing we do is weigh ourselves on electronic scales while answering questions on the attached iPads.

On a scale of one to five, where one is very bad and five is very good, how did you sleep?

One.

Why did you sleep so badly? Noise? Illness? Anxiety? Other.

Other.

Please elaborate.

Lyds saw a ghost.

The responses go straight to the conditioning team. You've never seen them move so fast. They're over at our table almost before we've sat down.

'What the hell's going on?'

When we turn in tonight, I take a sleeping tablet. I don't normally, but we're playing England tomorrow and I can't afford a third broken night's sleep. It's an evening match, kick-off 8.00 pm, so even if the pill does make me a bit lethargic first thing, it'll have cleared long before then.

Saturday, 26 September. I've played in a World Cup semi-final. I've played in Grand Slam deciders. I've played in Lions Tests. And none of them have been as hyped as this game has. It might 'only' be a pool match in the World Cup, but we all know it's much, much more than that.

We're each coming off the back of a win in our opening matches: England against Fiji, us against Uruguay. A lot of the press attention has been focused on England's selection of Sam Burgess at 12 – a rugby league great, certainly, but inexperienced and relatively untried at this level in union. This is only his second cap. He'll be facing Jamie, and some boffins have worked out that the impact of those two running into each other at full speed is the same as a 45 mph car crash.

We go into our changing-room. It's very hot, way more than it should be. It feels like a deliberate trick, something designed to make us lethargic; not from the England camp themselves, of course, but one of the Twickenham staff taking it upon themselves to try and mess with our heads. One of our management team goes off to sort it out.

Now the lights go off. This really is taking the piss. What's more, it's stupid. Whatever the person doing this is hoping to achieve, they're only going to succeed in doing the exact opposite. The more they try to put us off our stride, the more they try to unsettle and wind us up, the more focused and determined we're going to be.

I love playing at Twickenham anyway. Outside of the Millennium, it's my favourite stadium to play in. When I hear people talking about it not having much of an atmosphere and being full of corporate types who don't know one end of a rugby ball from another, I honestly think they must be talking about a totally different place. Sure, I only ever come here with Wales, and there's always an extra spice to any Wales–England match, but every crowd I've ever played in front of here has been exactly what a rugby crowd should be: passionate, partisan, hostile, committed.

The atmosphere isn't quite Millennium 2013, but it's not far off. We come out into a narrow strip of light on halfway, with the rest of the stadium lights dimmed just for the moment. There's not an empty seat in the house.

We're really, really up for this one. World Cup schedules can be as hectic and unforgiving as Lions tours, packing too many games into too short a timeframe, but in both cases you forget all about that for nights like this one. Nothing masks pain and fatigue like the adrenaline of a huge occasion.

First blood to us on three minutes. Courtney Lawes pulls a maul down and Dan kicks the penalty. They're level 10 minutes later, Farrell making a difficult kick – 45 metres out and on the angle – look easy.

Dan has a kick almost as hard, and makes it look almost as easy: 6–3. England coming at us, but we're competing well and slowing the ball down effectively. Farrell goes back into the pocket and drops for goal from 40 metres out. It's not the sweetest kick he's ever struck, but it goes over and we're back level.

Not much in this. Not much at all.

Tom Wood comes short off 9. Lyds goes so low he's practically eating grass and chops Wood, who goes flying over the top of him and spins 180 degrees in the air. The England lads are all around Lyds as he gets up, four or five of them in his face, and I barge my way in between them to get to him. No way am I leaving my mate undefended here, not in the heart of enemy country. There are a dozen blokes involved now, pushing and shoving.

There's a tug on my collar. I ignore it. Another, and again I ignore it. The third time it happens, hard enough to pull me off balance, I turn round to see what's going on. It's Brown, chopsing off at me. Scott Williams and Jamie are here now too, and more boys on both sides are piling in, and I'm laughing in Brown's face.

'What are you doing?' I say. 'You'd better leave quick before I catch you on your own later in the game.' On the commentary, Shane Williams is trying not to laugh. 'What's Mike Brown doing there, starting on an openside?' Brown then starts chopsing off at Gethin, who'd batter him even quicker than I would.

Lyds's tackle looked much worse than it actually was. The replay clearly shows Lyds leading with his right arm, as he's supposed to. Jérôme Garcès awards England the scrum, as they were in possession, and calls me and Chris Robshaw in. 'The scuffle afterwards, it's not necessary. I am in charge. We are in charge, the referees. I don't need your help, OK? Keep focused on your game.'

England get the better of us at the scrum, and are awarded the penalty when we drop it. On the 22, bang in front. Farrell's not going to miss this in a month of Sundays: 9–6 to England, the first time they've been ahead in the match.

They keep the pressure up. Lyds is pinged for holding on, Farrell finds touch just inside our 22, and from the lineout England work it across the field and through the phases. Anthony Watson comes off his wing and tries to feed Mike Brown. The pass goes to ground. England have numbers and recycle quickly for Youngs to put Johnny May over in the corner. Farrell adds the conversion, and in what seems a trice we've gone from three points up to ten points down.

If we go in like that at half-time, we'll be looking down the barrel of a gun. We press and press, but England hold firm and come back at us. Two minutes until the break and we put it through the hands to Scott Williams, who cuts through the England defence into the 22 and forces Brown to concede the penalty at the ruck, right in front of the posts. Dan nails it.

It's 16–9 to England at half-time. That kick felt worth more than three points.

Farrell and Dan trade penalties: 19–9, 19–12, 22–12, 22–15, 22–18. We're inching back into this, little by little, whittling away at England's buffer, making them worry about us rather than playing their own game. George gets away down the right and Liam takes it on.

Into the last quarter. Scott's knee goes in a tackle and he's stretchered off. Cuthie comes on and George shifts to 13.

Suddenly it's like a field hospital out there. Hallam Amos and Liam both have to go off too, replaced by Lloyd Williams and Rhys Priestland. Lloyd's a scrum-half, but he'll have to fill in on the wing for the last 14 minutes.

If we win from here, it'll rank up there with the best comebacks ever.

England are stretching us, looking to attack a backline in which half the guys are playing out of position. We have to smother it by fair means or foul. Coming-in-at-the-side foul, in fact: 25–18 to England with ten to go.

We need something. Anything.

Through the hands we go again. George has it, but May wraps him up. We go left. Jamie feeds Lloyd with very little to work with down the touchline. Brown giving him the outside, Watson covering back with Robshaw. Toby points to the inside. Lloyd drops the ball onto his left foot and kicks through and across, a hit-and-hope grubber; there are white shirts all around and only one red one, Gareth Davies, hammering up the middle more in hope than expectation, because no cause is lost until you give up on it.

The ball bounces: once, twice, three, four, five times, inching closer to the posts. Richard Wrigglesworth, bandage round his head, is turning to follow it, and May's there too with James Haskell, but Gareth's the one who's read it the best, Gareth's the one scooping it off his toes on the five-metre line and diving over under the posts as Wrigglesworth desperately tries to stop him.

Unbelievable. Just unbelievable. A lucky bounce? Sure. But you make your own luck in this game.

Dan converts: 25–25.

Minds on. Minds on. Next job.

Six minutes to go. Brown catches a high one on halfway. I'm jackalling on him like a fiend and he holds on. Garcès whistles. Penalty.

Dan hasn't missed all night. He's not going to start now: 28–25 to us.

Three minutes left. England have a lineout on our 22. They go right. Watson tries to get those quick, dancing feet of his going, but we shut the door on him. England send it back inside. Farrell comes round on the loop. Brown takes it up into contact. Once more I'm on him like a flash.

This is mine, sunshine. This is my turnover.

Garcès blows.

'Red 7, not releasing.'

I can't believe my ears. That was a legitimate jackal all day long.

Don't argue. The referee's word is law.

It's a tough ask, out near the touchline, but Farrell's been kicking well all night. A draw wouldn't be great, but it wouldn't be a disaster either, especially from where we've been for the last quarter of an hour with a patched-up backline.

Robshaw and George Ford have a quick conversation. Ford turns the ball over in his hands and sets his body away from the posts.

They're going for the corner. They're going for the corner, and the lineout, and the drive and the try, and that is an insult to every single player in a red jersey on this pitch. We don't think a draw's good enough, that's what England are saying. We don't think you've got it in you to hold us out.

Right. Bring it on. Bring it the f*** on.

Ford drills it into touch on our five-metre line. We set ourselves for the lineout while the England forwards take their time, walking slowly upfield, knowing this is their big chance, and wanting, needing, to get it right.

I march up and down our line like a sergeant major at Rorke's Drift. 'No way they get this! Stand your ground. Stand your f***ing ground! No one comes through here.'

I can hardly hear myself above the roar of the crowd.

They throw to Robshaw at the front. The moment I see him go up, I'm thinking that's a bonehead decision; it makes it way too easy for us to choke their maul off. They should be putting it to the middle or the back and trying to come through our midfield.

We don't even contest the jump. The moment Robshaw's feet touch the ground again we're piling in, swarming, shoving, grappling, a red tide driving them into touch.

Have some of that. F***ing have some of that.

Our lineout. Gareth Davies clears to touch, still inside our 22. Parling taps their lineout ball back but it's messy and Alun Wyn's first there to grab it. Gareth goes for another clearance kick, England charge it down, but Garcès calls us back for an England knock-on off the lineout ball.

Thirty seconds left. Gareth checks the call with Dan. England disrupt the scrum, but Toby scoops it up anyway and takes the contact. We form the ruck. Gareth looks up at the clock.

Seven seconds.

Garcès motioning for England to stay onside.

Three seconds.

Gareth whips it back to Dan in the in-goal area. Dan turns, waiting the last second or two for the clock to go red, and then boots it over the deadball line.

We've done it.

Just as I've never experienced hype like the anticipation around this game, so I've never experienced a changing-room atmosphere like this one afterwards. The sheer joy, the adrenaline of defiance and triumph: it's incredible. Beating England at the Millennium two years ago was amazing, but in some ways doing it at Twickenham has been even better – taking it to the enemy in the heart of their citadel, storming the ramparts of Fortress Twickenham. Two days ago it was Lyds who saw a ghost; now all the England boys look as if they're doing the same.

We crowd into the changing-room, not just the players but everyone involved in this campaign – the non-playing squad members, the management, the backroom staff – and we belt out 'Ar Lan y Môr' as loud as we can, so loud that we know England will hear it through the walls.

Ar lan y môr mae cerrig gleision
Ar lan y môr mae blodau'r meibion
Ar lan y môr mae pob rinweddau
Ar lan y môr mae nghariad innau.

Beside the sea blue pebbles lying
Beside the sea gold flowers glowing
Beside the sea are all things fairest
Beside the sea is found my dearest.

Robshaw is being pilloried in the media for his decision to go for the corner with three minutes left. I feel for him, and not just because he's a good bloke and my opposite number (both as captain and 7).

Was it the wrong decision? The obvious answer is yes, as it cost them at least a share of the match. Farrell had kicked six out of six from the tee plus a droppie, so he'd have been odds-on to nail that kick too and make it 28–28. But if Robshaw had gone for that he'd have been accused of bottling the chance of a win – a win that, with all the injuries we'd suffered, they perhaps felt should have been theirs anyway.

That's not a wrong decision other than how the result played out. If they'd gone for the corner and worked a try, he'd have been hailed as a genius. Even if we'd managed to hold them up, they'd have still had a good chance of the three points; they could have kept on with the phases either until we'd infringed or they'd worked Farrell in for another drop.

For me, the wrong decision England made in that play was not whether to kick for the corner or the three; it was to call the ball to the front of the lineout. That gave us the chance to do exactly what we did, which was steamroller them into touch and win the lineout ourselves. They should have gone to the middle or the back and taken us on in midfield. That they didn't do so wasn't just down to the captain, but to others too: the lineout caller, the pack leader and so on.

As I said in the 'Perspective' section, the captain never acts alone.

Saturday, 10 October. We're back at Twickenham for a match that few of the locals can be that thrilled about: us against Australia, knowing that we're both going through to the quarters come what may. England lost to Australia a week ago, while we beat Fiji, which was physically the hardest game I've ever played in; not just because it's always draining playing against such naturally strong and athletic men, but because it was our third match in 11 days and I was exhausted.

So all that's left to be decided is who wins the group and what that means for the quarter-final draw. The winner tonight will face Scotland, who only just squeaked through against Samoa this afternoon (if they'd lost, their place in the knockouts would have gone to Japan, who kickstarted this tournament on its second day with their once-in-a-lifetime victory over South Africa). The loser will face the Springboks, who overcame that shock defeat to top the group anyway.

We want Scotland, of course. No disrespect, but they'll be easier opponents. Not only are South Africa a better team, but we've beaten Scotland eight times in a row now, so we feel we have their number good and proper. I've never lost to them in my whole career so far. In contrast, our victory against South Africa last year was our first in 17 attempts. Win this match, get Scotland, and we'd be odds-on to at least match our semi-final run of four years ago.

We should do it. We should beat Australia. In the last quarter especially, we miss so many overlaps it's embarrassing. Justin and I nullify Pocock and Hooper at the breakdown, starving them of turnover ball. We spend long periods in their 22.

But – same old story – we can't quite close it out. That intensity we had against England just isn't there. Maybe it would be too much to expect us to peak again the way we had for that match. Maybe there's not quite the same do-or-die sword of Damocles hanging over you when you know you're through even if you lose. Whatever it is, they win 15–9, with no tries on either side.

South Africa it is, then.

Saturday, 17 October. I'm going out for the warm-up when there's a tap on my shoulder. It's Schalk Burger, who's playing blindside for the Springboks today.

He gestures to the ground, the crowd already beginning to fill up. 'This is awesome, eh? Let's just enjoy it.' It's typical not just of him but pretty much every South African I've ever played against. They're hard as nails on the pitch – not dirty, just incredibly physical – but off it they're the nicest people.

The match is a heavyweight slugfest, a proper old school Test: two very good sides going at it hammer and tongs, no quarter asked and none given. With six minutes to go, we're clinging on 19–18, but they have a scrum near the touchline on our 22.

The scrum wheels left towards the blindside. Duane Vermeulen picks up from the base and drives. Lloyd clings on to his ankles, and with the scrum now at almost 90 degrees I can't quite get to him, and Cuthie comes up off the blindside wing to help. Vermeulen waits until Cuthie's on him before flipping a no-look ball out of the back of his hand to Fourie du Preez on the loop, and du Preez dives in at the corner for the winning try. Heartbreaker.

After the match, the Springbok coach Heyneke Meyer hugs me and tells me what a great game it was. We're the first quarter-final, and in their own way they all turn out to be memorable: the All Blacks destroy France later in the evening, and the next day Argentina run it from everywhere to beat Ireland, and Scotland play out a rollercoaster thriller against Australia, which is only decided right at the end on a very contentious offside penalty – a decision that will have huge ramifications two years from now, though of course none of us know that yet.

We're out, but we couldn't have given anything more. And in all honesty even if we had won, I couldn't have played the semi as I'm just so battered. I don't have any one specific bad injury, just a series of grade 1s all over my body.

And I'm not the only one. Our injury list is so long that in a way I'm glad we didn't make it through; we'd have had to send out a largely young and inexperienced team against an All Blacks side at the top of their game, and a heavy defeat would have left that team with mental scars that would have taken a long time to heal.

I've never been the kind of player to think that beating England is or should be the be-all and end-all of Welsh ambitions. But if that victory at Twickenham ended up as being the high water mark of this campaign – well, there are worse memories to have.

Saturday, 28 November. I do my ankle ligament colliding with Tips, of all people, in a match against the Ospreys. Two months out. Injury #18.

Sunday, 7 February 2016. We claw back a 13-point deficit against Ireland in the opening round of the Six Nations to draw 16–16. I'm playing opposite CJ Stander, but I don't realise until the post-match dinner that this was his debut. When someone tells me, I go to get my shirt and give it to him. He offers his back, of course, but I say no, you must keep it: you only ever make your debut once.

Saturday, 12 March. I'm knocked unconscious while playing against England at Twickenham. It's a complete accident – in fact, it's Alun Wyn who clips me rather than one of the England players – but the medics are taking no chances. They put me in a neck brace and carry me off on a stretcher. I give a thumbs-up to the crowd to let them know I'm OK, but I only know this afterwards when I'm shown the footage: I have no awareness of it at the time.

When I come round in the medics' room, I'm desperate to find my phone and let everyone know I'm OK. It's all right, the medics say. We've already spoken to your wife and let her know you're fine.

Injury #19.

We score two tries in the last six minutes, but we've left ourselves too much ground to make up. England hang on to win 25–21.

Sunday, 13 March. Dad is walking his dog when a woman stops him.

'How on earth did we lose that yesterday?' she says.

He mumbles something non-committal, hoping that will end the conversation, but she keeps going. 'We should have beaten them, we should have …'

'I don't give a shit!' Dad snaps. 'When your son's put in a neck brace and carried off on a stretcher, the result's the last thing you care about, you know?'

Dad never snaps at people, never loses his temper like that. It's a sign of how much he and Mum are worried about me; not just for the incident yesterday, but for all the ones that have come before and all the ones that might happen in the future.

Always play for Wales as though it's your last game, Gats keeps saying. One day it will be.

'How long are you going to keep playing for?' Mum asks.

Saturday, 30 April. I sprain the ACJ in my right shoulder. The medics reckon I'll just about make it back in time for the summer tour of New Zealand. Injury #20.

Thursday, 14 July. Rach gives birth to a beautiful baby girl, Anna Victoria Kennedy-Warburton. She weighs – of course – 7 lb.

She might have my number, but luckily she doesn't have my nose.

Saturday, 1 October. I fracture my cheekbone in a clash of heads with Leinster's Josh van der Flier and need surgery to have a plate inserted. Injury #21.

Saturday, 26 November. I sit out the autumn international against South Africa after getting a stinger in training earlier in the week. It's a shame, because the WRU have made the match a bit special for us. They've asked each squad member to invite someone who made a difference to us in our early days: a teacher, a club coach, a family member, anyone without whom we might not have developed a love of rugby.

It's a lovely idea, and shows the importance of rugby in our lives both and off the pitch. Dan Biggar and Sam Davies have both nominated their former geography teacher Dean Mason, who says that 'rugby is not about the person who becomes an international, it's about how rugby develops other skills too, raises self-esteem, improves personal and interpersonal skills. We want to develop the best rugby players we can but also the best citizens we can. As a teacher you want to try to inspire people to be the best they can be at whatever they are, and personally I'm more proud of Dan and Sam as fantastic young men and role models than of what they are achieving on the rugby field.'

I've asked Frank Rees, my old headmaster at Llanishen Fach who made me play rugby all those years ago because he saw how good I could be. Without him, who knows how different my life might have been?

I think of all the people here today, all these men and women who've given us so much, who one day saw a spark in a child and fanned that spark until it caught fire and spread and blossomed and consumed that child's life.

And I think that this must surely be the holy grail of teaching. Not exam results or league tables, but being the one who actually makes a difference to a child's life, who helps them achieve their potential or saves them from disaster. When the endless paperwork swamps you and the constant pressure gets you down, that must be the light in the darkness: the adult who knows that without what you did for them as a child, they wouldn't be who and what they are today.

Monday, 26 December. It's my 100th game for the Blues, and I get a box for the whole family to come and watch – including baby Anna, who sees her dad play for the first time. It's an emotional day for me, notching up this milestone for the only professional club I've ever played for. Even though a combination of central contracts and injuries have meant that my appearances for the Blues are restricted, I hope the fans know how much this means to me. We beat the Dragons 27–16, which is a nice way to mark it.

Sunday, 5 February 2017. Our opening Six Nations game, against Italy. Alun Wyn is captain, a decision that I'm totally on board with. Over the past few months I've been talking to Rob Howley about it on and off, and we've both decided that I'd be better off without the captaincy. I just want to concentrate on my own game again.

And the reason it's Rob I've been talking to rather than Gats is also the reason I want to concentrate on my own game. Gats is away on Lions duty again, and I want to give myself the best chance possible of making that plane.

Monday, 13 February. Our first analysis meeting after losing to England on Saturday, a match we should have won. A lot of the match reports are pointing the finger at Foxy, whose failure to find touch with a clearance kick allowed England to run the ball back at us and score what turned out to be the winning try.

I put my hand up. Yes, I said, Foxy shanked the kick; but why did he need to take that kick in the first place? That was because of a mistake I made a few minutes earlier. We had an attacking lineout in their half, and Jake Ball called a move that involved me lifting at the back. I misunderstood the call, and for some reason thought we didn't have the option Jake was calling when in fact we did. It was my brain fart, not Jake's. I didn't lift the man when I should have done, which meant that the ball was overthrown, that England got possession and worked their way into the position where Foxy was forced to try to clear our lines in a hurry.

If I'd done my job, we'd have won that match.

The coaches know all this, of course, and if I didn't own up they'd have presented me with the evidence in front of the whole team. What they wanted to see, and what I've done, is me being honest enough to take ownership of my mistake.

Friday, 7 April. The Blues are playing away in Ulster. The Six Nations is done and dusted, and though Wales didn't do too well – we came fifth, having won two and lost three – I felt it was personally the best Six Nations I'd played since 2011. I'm on good form and not worried about being picked for the Lions. Even though I haven't spoken to Gats in a while, I know enough about the way I'm playing, and the way he likes to think, to be as sure as I can be that I'm on that plane.

I'm walking back in from the warm-up with Rory Best who, like me, is often mentioned as a potential Lions captain. The squad's due to be announced in 12 days' time.

'You heard anything?' we ask each other pretty much simultaneously.

Neither of us have. I wonder who else is in the frame. Alun Wyn, possibly, and maybe also Johnny Sexton, though I know Gats prefers to have a forward as captain if possible.

Today's match is a bit of a non-event for us: we can't reach the play-offs, though Ulster still can. With the Lions in mind, it's really important that I don't get injured.

I get injured.

I'm standing up out of a ruck when I take a hit. There's a shooting pain in my knee that I try to run off, but when I change direction I know it's more than a tweak. The physio comes on.

'It's a grade 2 ligament strain,' I tell him. I know my own body and its injury list so well by now that I can do my own diagnosis.

'Off you come,' he says. If this were a cup final with no summer tour ahead, I'd risk carrying on, but another nudge would turn it into a grade 3 and that would be my Lions tour over.

Six weeks out. I'll still make the tour, but I'll have to work hard to get up to match fitness in time for the Test matches. Injury #22.

Not everyone thinks I should be skipper. Under the headline **LIONS STAND NO CHANCE OF UPSET IF WARBURTON IS GIVEN CAPTAINCY**, Stuart Barnes writes in *The Times* that 'the odds are against the Lions winning the series in New Zealand. They will grow even greater should Warburton once again be named their leader. He would make a magnificent midweek leader. But not the Test team. He doesn't possess that extra ingredient [needed to beat New Zealand].'

Thursday, 13 April. I'm in the car with Rach. We pull into the Sainsbury's car park. I clear my throat. 'I don't want to look like one of those lazy husbands who makes their wife do all the chores ...'

'... but you'd like to me to go in and do the shopping on my own.' Rach finishes the sentence for me.

'Please.'

She knows why I'm asking: because if I go in with her we're going to have two dozen people ask me if I've heard about the Lions captaincy yet, and I just can't be bothered with that. I've had it every day for about a month now. Perhaps I should have got a T-shirt made up.

NO, I HAVEN'T SPOKEN TO WARREN GATLAND.

NO, I DON'T KNOW IF I'M LIONS CAPTAIN.

NO, I WOULDN'T TELL YOU EVEN IF I DID KNOW.

But I *do* want the captaincy. I really want it. In 2013 I wasn't really expecting it, and I doubted whether I was up to it. I've been through a lot since then. I'm older, harder, tougher. Forged. I want Gats to ring, and I want him to ask me, because at some deep level this is what I feel my career has been building to all along, the keeping of the promise I made to myself when I got back from Sydney four years ago.

Rach goes into the supermarket. I keep my head down so I don't get buttonholed by someone walking past the car and seeing that I'm inside.

My phone rings. **GATS.** Here we go.

A bit of small talk: how was the Ulster game, how's your injury, how's the recovery coming along? Not bad, not bad, not bad to all three.

'I was just wondering, Warby, do you want to be Lions captain again?'

'Mate, definitely. Damn right I'll be captain.'

LEADERSHIP 6: PERSISTENCE

No leader is perfect, no matter how good they think they are. Every leader always has room for improvement, no matter how minuscule they feel that improvement may be. Accepting the first and pursuing the second come down to the same thing: persistence.

It took me three or four years until I felt I was a good captain. At the 2011 World Cup, during the 2012 Grand Slam, even on the 2013 Lions tour, I felt the same thing: there were others in those sides who could do the job better than I could. It wasn't until round about 2014 or 2015 that I felt deep down that I now belonged in the job.

Perhaps it was because I'd been doing it for a while by then, perhaps it was (a little perversely) because of an internal challenge to my leadership around that time, perhaps it was because my professional and personal lives had both moved on to permanent footings with a central contract and marriage respectively. Perhaps it was all of these, or some, or none. It doesn't really matter.

What matters is that I'd kept on at it. I'd kept on at making myself a better leader, through all the times I'd doubted myself, until I finally felt I was worth the role that I perhaps hadn't felt myself worth when I'd first been given it. Only with the hindsight that persistence brought me could I see how much I'd have regretted turning it down in 2011. Smiler had told me as much when he phoned me before the World Cup that year, and he'd been right.

Persistence as a leader involves constant self-questioning. If you do something well, can you do it even better? If you don't do something so well, how can you improve that? I'd refer to the leadership compass that Andy and I had drawn up during the 2011 World Cup, and assess as honestly as I could how I was doing in each of the four areas on that compass: professional attitude, positive attitude, my own performance and leading by example, and developing personal relationships with the players.

Professional attitude. I always prided myself on being the most professional member of any squad I played in. The greater the number of my team-mates who aspired to that level the better, both from a collective point of view (team standards were improving) and an individual one too (if I wanted to maintain my position as the most professional member, I had to keep improving my standards too). At international level, professionalism isn't drinking nine pints a night when everyone else is having ten; it's forever seeking little advantages in training, recovery, nutrition and so on.

Positive attitude. For the most part, this also came easily to me. I'm a positive person, and what Gats had identified in that clip of me with Josh Turnbull in the 2011 match against England wasn't something I had to force. But equally there were plenty of times when I wasn't feeling that positive: when I was tired of the pressure, or the injuries, or some of the internal politicking. When that was the case, I always tried to keep my negativity to myself, or share it only with a very few people whom I trusted. In a team environment, both positivity and negativity emanate more from the person at the top than from any other single person, and they're both contagious. Positivity's worth catching. Negativity isn't.

My own performance. You can't always work harder – no matter how fit and strong you are, there's a limit to how much the human body can take – but you can work smarter. For the first few years of my professional career, I'd look at my stats without questioning too much below the raw numbers. Turnovers secured, rucks hit, tackles made, metres carried: all pretty self-explanatory, right?

Not quite. There's no point in hitting 50 rucks a game, for example, if you're not being effective at most of those rucks – if your body position's wrong, or if your side has enough players there already for you not to make a difference. In those circumstances, you'd be better off taking up your position in the defensive line.

Similarly, a bare '20 tackles made' doesn't say how important those tackles were, how many drove the tackled player backwards, how many led to a knock-on or similar; and 'metres made' doesn't show the speed at which those metres were made, or the angles, or the space created by those runs.

By the end of my career, I was playing far smarter than at the beginning, knowing that raw numbers don't tell the full story. Against Italy during the 2017 Six Nations, for instance, I was involved in only 20 rucks, but I was effective – that is, my presence was essential to the ball being won – at 15 of them, a strike rate of 75 per cent. Working harder? No. Working smarter? Definitely.

Developing personal relationships with the players. This was definitely my weak spot to begin with, and the one I had to show most persistence in improving. As I got to know the boys better – and it helped that the nucleus of our team was settled over several years, so this process became easier and more organic than it would have been with an endlessly revolving door of personnel – I became better at sensing the group's mood and working with that.

Part of learning to be a better leader is to be flexible within certain parameters. If people say they're tired and want a rest, are they just being lazy or do they feel it would be beneficial in the long run? I couldn't answer this question without knowing the boys well enough to understand their baseline moods.

There was one occasion when Toby Faletau said, almost as a throwaway line, that he was tired. Now, Toby never gets tired and he never complains; so when he says something like that, it's a sure sign that you need to think about making some changes, if only temporarily.

A similar thing happened, but on a larger scale, before the 2015 World Cup. We'd booked a training block in Spala, the Polish resort where we'd had such a productive camp before the 2011 World Cup. In 2015, however, we'd already been to Switzerland and Qatar, and the boys felt as though a third session abroad was too much, and that we could do the same amount of work at our usual Vale resort in Wales without the hassle of travelling.

I had to assess the mood. This feeling was clearly pretty widespread, and the commitment the boys had shown in Switzerland and Qatar had been exemplary. Added to that, the nucleus of players I mentioned now had several years' experience and a good number of caps. Whatever they were, they weren't shirkers.

So I went to talk to the management team. They weren't happy about this, not least because Spala had been booked and paid for, and the WRU stood to lose a lot of money if we didn't go and used the Vale instead. But I ran through my arguments clearly and consistently, and pointed out that all we were trying to do was maximise our chances of getting to the knockout stages – and if we did then the WRU would recoup the lost money many times over.

It was in some ways the hardest thing I ever did as captain, and I know there's no way that I'd have had the balls to do it in the first year or two I was skipper. Because it wasn't just about the money, of course. It was effectively the players saying to Gats, 'On this issue, we know better than you' – which was a difficult message to convey to one of the best coaches in the world, a man for whom I had the utmost respect and without whom I might well not have captained either Wales or the Lions.

But I had to do it. And the management team listened, and in the end they accepted it, not least because my relentless determination to consistently make myself a better player and leader had earned me enough credit to be taken seriously. I walked back into the team room, and everyone was going, 'Warby, I bet you bottled it.' I just stood there like Leonardo DiCaprio in *The Wolf of Wall*

Street with my arms out wide and said, 'Boys, we're not going to Poland.' You could have heard the cheers in Neath.

As this shows, the learning process also applied to my relationship with the coaches. As I got to know them better and felt more secure in my position, I began to question them more, and I realised that they wanted me to do this; they wanted to be pushed and to be challenged, because they wanted to keep improving as coaches just as I wanted to keep improving as a captain and player.

For instance, at the 2011 World Cup, Gats took me off with just under ten minutes to go in the pool match against Fiji. We had no subs left to bring on, I wasn't hurt, and he didn't tell the other players; he just wanted to see how they'd adapt to playing with 14 men. We were winning 59–0 at the time, so the match was long settled. In the remaining minutes, the players did just what he wanted them to do: defended our line superbly and scored a try at the other end.

It doesn't just have to be the captain or the coach who shows persistence. Anyone can do it, and in doing so it lifts the spirits and the standards. Take Pence in training. He was an amazing trainer. He'd always push himself 100 per cent, when most of the boys would be going around 90 per cent and trying to save a bit just in case.

There was one training session we did for the Blues on the Merthyr Mawr sand dunes outside Bridgend. The concept was simple: the entire squad raced up the highest, hardest dune. Whoever won that race, his session was over; everyone else went down to the bottom and started again. So it was quite tactical.

You had to work out on which round you had the best chance of winning and save your best effort for that one without emptying your tank too early.

Anyway, Pence was as quick and fit as a butcher's dog, so he fancied his chances of winning the very first round, when everyone was still in the frame, and then lounging around for the rest of the session giving us some abuse. He went hell for leather on that first one, but narrowly lost. Then he went hell for leather on the second one, and narrowly lost that too. By the time the third rep came round he was suffering. The fourth one was between me and him, and I beat him. Now he coasted for a couple of rounds, just to get his breath back, but he was so knackered that he still couldn't close any of the rounds out when he ramped it up to maximum again. Eventually there were just two men left: him, and a big prop called Salesi Ma'afu. And Ma'afu beat him!

On the face of it, Pence came last. But actually you could argue that he won, because he went hardest and never gave up. His persistence was awesome to behold. Someone said, 'How can he be the best trainer when he came last?' and I replied, 'He came last *because* he's the best trainer.'

It was a great lesson for all of us. It's tough to be persistent, and it takes persistence to be tough. Being tough isn't belting someone behind the ref's back; it's never giving up, it's always wanting the ball even when you're having a shit game, it's about getting up one more time than you're knocked down. It's about never settling for second best, and never settling for what you are today, because tomorrow you could be better.

7

WESTPAC STADIUM, WELLINGTON

41.2729°S, 174.7859°E

Saturday, 1 July 2017. British and Irish Lions v New Zealand, Second Test

Sonny Bill Williams drops his arms and shoulder-charges Anthony Watson straight in the face. The crowd gasp. Jérôme Garcès blows his whistle. Anthony's down on his knees, groggy from the hit.

'Warby!' Faz shouts. 'Speak to the ref! Shoulder to head's a straight red!'

I look at Garcès. He's already talking to the TMO, so I know they're going to have a look. That's all I need to know. No point spending my chips on this one. If the hit's as bad as it looked, Garcès will see that and he'll make the right decision. If it's not, no amount of me getting in his face will make a difference.

I turn back to Faz. 'Mate, leave it. They're taking a look.'

The replay comes up on the big screen. You can see the fear in Anthony's eyes in the last half-second before the impact, when he knows what's coming and tries to duck his face away. Every time the hit's shown and Anthony's head snaps back the crowd wince, and the Lions fans are booing and whistling, because it looks more and more like a straight red each time.

No referee has ever sent an All Black off in a Test on New Zealand soil.

I'd better have got this right.

Four years ago, I thought captaining the Lions was the ultimate. Now I realise that it wasn't. Captaining the Lions in New Zealand, the most iconic rugby nation on earth, isn't even the ultimate. Captaining the Lions to a series victory in New Zealand: *that* would be the ultimate.

What will I do to beat New Zealand? Whatever it takes.

It was this tour 12 years ago that first really fired my interest in the Lions. I immersed myself in that tour, getting up at stupid o'clock to watch some of the games. Martyn Williams was my hero, and I was so thrilled when he made it onto the pitch as a replacement in the third Test, even though the match and the series were long gone by then. I was also transfixed by the way Marty Holah played for the Maori All Blacks when they beat the Lions before the Test series began.

That tour was a disaster for the Lions, though; whitewashed 3–0 in the Tests, the squad split into two, and full of tensions off the pitch. Even the New Zealand public were disappointed, since they wanted a good, hard contest as much as anyone else. It's up to us to erase the memories of that tour and ensure that when New Zealanders come to remember the 2017 Lions, they do so with awe rather than disdain, with respect rather than pity.

No one gives us a chance. Of course they don't. In the black corner are the back-to-back world champions who've managed to replace four all-time greats – McCaw, Dan Carter, Ma'a Nonu and Conrad Smith – in the two years since the 2015 World Cup without missing a beat. In the red corner are a scratch side drawn from four different countries who will have less than six weeks between their first training session and the start of the Test series.

'It's not arrogance,' former All Black fly-half Nick Evans writes in the *Guardian*, 'but New Zealanders are expecting a 10–0 sweep of the Lions.' That's expecting the pick of the Home Nations to lose not just to the All Blacks but to every Super Rugby franchise too, plus the Maori All Blacks and the Provincial Barbarians. Every Lions side since the war has won at least half their tour matches, and usually a much higher proportion than that.

In fairness, Nick's speaking for the New Zealand public rather than himself. He personally doesn't think we'll lose many, if any, of the non-Test games, but he does think the Tests will be 3–0 to the All Blacks. Most pundits are saying similar things, perhaps conceding that we might win the final Test as a dead rubber once the series has gone, much as the 2009 Lions did in South Africa.

The number of people who think we can even take it to the final weekend is pretty small. The number who think we can win the series is detectable only by electron microscope. The bookies have New Zealand as 2/7 for the series, and though I don't know any more about betting than I did four years ago, people tell me those odds are close to a dead cert in a two-horse race.

I've never thought I'm going to lose an international match, and I'm certainly not going to start now.

Monday, 8 May. Messy Monday, when all the boys first meet up at Syon Park. I see Ben Te'o, and remember I've got a bone to pick with him about the time he fractured my cheekbone two years ago.

Rather annoyingly, he turns out to be a great bloke.

Gats gives us a form to fill in that includes questions like, 'How did you feel when you were named in the squad?', 'What are you going to bring to the squad?', 'List five strengths about you as a player,' that kind of stuff, all connected to positive affirmation.

He also decides we're going to have a choir; that singing is going to be part of the tour and that it will help us bond. The Welsh lads, of course, don't need a second invitation. They don't even need a second pint. But the English, the Irish and the Scots are less keen.

Gats is determined. We agree that we'll have four songs. Each country can choose their song and have a representative responsible for making everyone learn that song. So for Wales it's 'Calon Lân', led by Ken Owens; the English have 'Jerusalem' and Kyle Sinckler; the Irish go for 'Fields of Athenry', led by Robbie Henshaw; and the Scots have 'Highland Cathedral' and Greig Laidlaw.

Every night after training in the Vale, we have half an hour's choir practice with Haydn James, the Welsh choirmaster who does the games at the Principality Stadium. To start with, very few of the boys want to put their heads above the parapet, but gradually people get more into it. 'You all have to know the words by the time we land in New Zealand,' Gats says. 'We'll be singing them on live TV, and no one's going to be able to stand at the back and blag it.'

Sinks is already taking on the role of tour hero: the squad joker, the central point of all the banter and abuse, just like Hibbs had been in 2013. One day, while playing table tennis, he dives for a ball that anyone else would have let go – there's no way he's going to get there, but he's so competitive that he tries anyway – and the table collapses beneath him. He's lying there like a beached whale, and everyone's absolutely killing themselves laughing, him most of all.

Friday, 26 May. On our last night in Dublin, we all go out for a squad piss-up. Suddenly Sinks leaps up on a table and starts belting out 'Jerusalem'. It's not much more than a bar or two later that we all join in. It's tuneless but heartfelt, and the other punters in the place are loving it as much as we are.

After 'Jerusalem' we sing the other three songs with equal gusto; no lyric sheets, no song books. It turns out that the boys really have been learning the words properly, and have properly bought into the whole thing. What I thought might be an embarrassment has ended up galvanising the group.

The whole night is brilliant. You can do all the training and bonding exercises in the world, but sometimes nothing brings people together like a piss-up. Some of the quietest boys really come out of their shells once they have an ale or two inside them, and I know that tomorrow there'll be gales of laughter from people re-living the night before.

I buy myself a second mobile phone. The only people who'll have this number are my team-mates, family and close friends. My usual phone I'm switching off for the duration of the tour. I'm getting rid of all distractions, anything extraneous and unimportant. It's what Andy's been drumming into me for years – just say no. The next six weeks are all Lions, nothing else; a little bubble with my eyes always, always, on the prize.

Just as I did before the 2013 tour, I go for a walk with Andy. We go to The Wenallt, a local beauty spot that is a riot of bluebells in the spring. He takes me through a relaxation session here, and just as before tells me that whenever things get stressful on tour, I should take myself back here in my head.

Thursday, 1 June. From the moment we land in New Zealand, we have five security guys with us. They're all ex-military, either Special Forces or Marines, and they're very patient in answering over and again the two questions they get asked most often: how many people have you killed, and how realistic is *Call of Duty*?

Whenever there's a night out, they're the ones who take us there in the Lions-branded Land Rovers – having reconnoitred the place in advance – and they're the ones who ensure there's no trouble. We all know that they're in charge, no matter how much bigger than them any of us might be. If someone's got too merry and the security guys say they're taking him home, that lad has two choices: do what he's told or be a human pretzel on the floor.

Sometimes we see them relaxing in the team room, but there'll only ever be two of them in there at once. The others will be patrolling the hotel, or scoping out the next training ground to ensure that all the security cameras are turned off and that there are no hidden cameras in the hospitality boxes; both of those, of course, so that our sessions can't be filmed.

Most of the boys don't notice any of this, which is the way it should be. But make no mistake, the security guys keep the show on the road just as much as the coaches and the support staff do.

Saturday, 3 June. In Whangarei for the opening match of the tour. We squeak home against the Provincial Barbarians 13–7, and immediately the press are into us: these guys are semi-pro, why aren't you sticking 50 points on them?

Well, we're not sticking 50 points on them because this is a game we're totally ill-prepared for and which we should never have played. In my end-of-tour meeting with Charlie McEwen, the Lions' chief operating officer, this will be the very first thing I bring up.

We've only been in New Zealand a couple of days. Everyone's jetlagged and feeling lethargic. The atmosphere in the changing-room pre-match is flat, way off the usual levels of anticipation. Some of the boys even doze off on the way to the game. That should never happen, not at any kind of professional level.

Either we should have come over much earlier – a week beforehand, minimum – and given ourselves time to acclimatise, or we shouldn't have played the game in the first place, which would have been my preference. We're on a hiding to nothing: if we win it's expected, if we lose it's a disaster. We don't need it at the end of a long season, and it will make no difference to the selection of the Test team.

Besides, semi-pro in New Zealand is a totally different kettle of fish than it is in other countries. It's not like when we played the Combined County team in Australia four years ago. The Provincial Barbarians are a good side, not that far off Super Rugby standards, and if I'd been scouting for a top European club side I'd have been in the stands today taking some serious interest in some of the players on show.

Wednesday, 7 June. Auckland. We play the Blues, the first and weakest of the five Super Rugby franchises on our itinerary. They haven't beaten another Kiwi franchise all season. Even though you'd think relatively few members of the side today will make the Test team, we really should do them over.

We don't.

We go down 22–16, courtesy of a brilliant Ihaia West try with five minutes to go. Even then we have chances to snatch the win, but we concede a penalty when we don't need to and then botch a lineout. There are positives – our scrum goes well, our line speed in D is good – but we don't offer much by way of penetration, and the Blues defence finds it relatively easy to drift across and use the touchline as a shadow.

A loss today isn't the end of the world. But this will have given New Zealand rugby a taste of blood, and like sharks the other teams will fancy getting themselves a piece as well –

starting on Saturday in Christchurch, when we're facing the best Super Rugby team of all, the Crusaders.

I hear a lovely story afterwards, the kind of story you only get on Lions tours. A Lions supporter called Alex Edwards turned up at Ponsonby Rugby Club in his campervan, hoping to park up and sleep there. A woman called Sandra Wihongi said he could come and stay in her house if he liked. So he did, and had a cup of tea and a chat with her two adult sons when they turned up. After they'd gone, he said, 'Your lads must play to a decent standard, being that big.' Turns out they were Rieko and Akira Ioane, who were playing for the Blues against us.

Everywhere we go, we hear this kind of thing: locals who bring Lions fans into their houses, lend them their cars to drive around in, and so on. This is the kind of country not just where a hotel chambermaid can tell you that your body position at the ruck is wrong, but also where she'll be spot on.

Rugby binds everyone together, and for all the guys you get who'll come up and say, 'You've got no chance,' there are many, many more who are totally lovely and just thrilled that the Lions are here. Everywhere the Lions bus goes, people will cheer and take pictures. In Australia there were times when we could go more or less incognito. Not here. Not for one moment.

Thursday, 8 June. 'There's a poll been taken of 200 people in Auckland,' says a reporter at a press conference, 'asking them to name three players in this Lions squad, and only five people managed it. What does that tell you?'

I half-laugh, giving myself a few seconds to think about what to say.

First rule of professional sport: never give the opposition's team talk for them. That's what this reporter is doing, whether she means to or not. There are 45 of the most competitive men you'll ever meet on this tour, so whatever psychology you think you're using isn't going to work. But I'm not going to bite, even though what I really want to say is, 'I couldn't give a toss about your stupid survey.'

Before I can answer, Gats jumps in and says something nice and diplomatic.

At training in the afternoon, I'm sitting in the stands with Mako Vunipola, and I tell him what this reporter said. Mako's got the most expressive eyebrows since Roger Moore, and he raises one of them just a fraction now.

'They'll know who we are when we smash 'em on Saturday, won't they?' he says.

That evening a few of us go to the Memorial Wall, which commemorates those who died in the Christchurch earthquake six years ago. Gats has mates who are engineers here, and apparently there are still some places that are uninhabitable because of aftershocks. The Crusaders are clearly really important to this city during its reconstruction, and their blazing start to the season – 14 wins out of 14, an average of 37 points per game – has given people a lift.

I meet a woman called Sarah O'Connor and her boys Dan and Sean, who must be around eight and six years of age. 'Come and see our dad,' they say. I think they're going to take me to meet one of the blokes in the crowd, but instead they take me to the Memorial Wall itself and show me his name: John O'Connor, one of 185 people killed in the earthquake.

It's all I can do to stop myself breaking down right here and now. These two lovely little lads, so proud of and full of love for their dad. I think about Anna back at home, not even a year old, and the thought of me leaving her behind and her growing up without me just finishes me, it really does.

They take me back to their mum. John was a mad keen Irish rugby fan, she explains, so he'd have been supporting us on Saturday.

'Are you going to the match?' I ask.

She shakes her head. 'It's a sell-out. We couldn't get tickets.'

'Can you give me a second?'

I go over to Charlie McEwen. 'Mate, these guys haven't got tickets. I can give the boys my two personal ones. Can you get one for Sarah too?'

'Course I can,' he says.

Saturday, 10 June. Gats has said that dropping a couple of games in the build-up to the Tests wouldn't be the end of the world, providing that we're still making progress as a squad. But sometimes you need a result too, to build momentum and self-belief. Tonight is one of those times.

We've put out what looks very much like a shadow Test side (though, in fact, 13 of the starters tonight will start the first Test). The Crusaders have got nine All Blacks in their ranks.

No more excuses, no more shadow boxing. For the first time this tour, this is the real deal. We have to beat them. We have to put down a marker. If we lose, that's two games out of three gone, defeats at the hands of both Super Rugby franchises we've played so far, and the tour might well be in freefall.

We're so much better than we were against the Blues. Our intensity and physicality are right up where they need to be, and there's an edge that wasn't there in Whangarei or Auckland. Conor and Faz boss the show tactically at half-back, our breakdown work is good and our defence suffocating. The final score is 12–3 to us, with no tries scored – the first time the Crusaders have failed to cross the line in more than two years – but both sides know the margin could have been more.

The entire squad comes into the changing-room after the match: smacking backs, hugging blokes, giving it the big celebrations. Someone shouts 'Sinks!' to lead the singing, and we pump out 'Highland Cathedral', really pump it out. A strong win, a big win, and the tour's back on course.

Some of the questions at the press conference accuse us of playing negative rugby. Gats is having none of it. 'It's only the third time in their history the Crusaders have scored only three points in a match and both of the other occasions were away from home. The [Lions] team that played tonight has been together for only a week, and this is the sixth hotel we've stayed in since we've been in New Zealand. We made 13 line breaks. I didn't see any negative rugby.'

There's a minor tremor (4.2 on the Richter scale) in the stadium after the conference. If we keep on improving, we've got a good chance of springing a bigger shock on everyone who thought this would be a whitewash.

As for the New Zealand public – they know who we are now, don't they?

Tuesday, 13 June. Dunedin. I've only played one match on this tour so far, just over an hour against the Provincial Barbarians before coming off as a precaution after an ankle strain. I need game time and I need it now.

As with the last midweek match against the Blues, we should win, and as with that match we don't. We're 22–13 up with 20 minutes to go, but in that last quarter they score ten points without reply to beat us by a point. Sure, we can moan about one penalty against Dan Cole that we all think should go the other way, and without that we'd have won, but those things are part of the game. We need more control and more accuracy than we show.

Once again we seem to be taking one step back for every two forward, losing at a time when we'd just started to build momentum again with the Crusaders win. But, to be brutal, the side we've put out is very much a midweek one – the gap between the Test starters and the rest is already pretty clear – and it shows. Only a couple of the boys tonight really press their claims for a Test spot.

I get 68 minutes, plus a try, to go with my 66 against the Provincial Barbarians. I haven't played badly in either match, but equally I haven't played outstandingly. I'll get better – I know I need four games to hit my straps and get the engine going, so two more games will sharpen me up – but right now on form alone I'm not first pick on either flank. Sean O'Brien's playing better than me at seven, and Peter O'Mahony likewise at six.

And it hurts. My body's not allowing me to do everything I want, and I want this – to captain the side to a series win – more than anything else. I can't afford to be off the pace.

'How are you feeling?' Gats says.

There's no point beating about the bush. 'I don't want to make the decision for you,' I reply, 'but I know I'm not at the level of the Six Nations yet. So I won't be upset not to be in the starting XV for the first Test.'

'That's very honest. I appreciate that.'

I've more or less deselected myself, which some people might find strange. But you can't preach about the team being the most important thing and then put your own individual needs above that. And I know I've got history on my side. I was a little rusty going into the 2013 tour, and it showed in the first Test, when I was still getting back to peak form; but in the second Test I played one of the games of my life.

Gats and I go back a long way as coach and captain: two Lions tours, two World Cups and eight regular seasons with Wales. If I can't be honest with him, who can I be honest with?

Saturday, 17 June. Rotorua. If the midweek team are going to keep losing, then the Saturday team have to keep winning. The Maori All Blacks promise to be even more of a challenge than the Crusaders were, and by the same token it's even more of a must-win match. We're only a week out from the first Test.

We don't win as well as we did against the Crusaders. We win better: 32–10, including a second-half shutout. 'As good a night as Gatland has enjoyed since the third Lions Test in Sydney four years ago,' one report says, and it's bang on. We dominate territory and possession, playing to the conditions (rainy enough to make even us Welshmen feel at home). We're defensively solid, and yet when the chances come we're being increasingly clinical when we take them. I come on with 16 minutes left, and even in that short time feel that I'm playing better than I did against the Highlanders.

The win's also a testament to the way the training sessions are being run. It doesn't matter how good you are individually, it takes time for combinations to build and teams to come together. Gats and the coaches are always on at us to do four things:

- Be more physical than anyone we face, which is pretty self-explanatory. Win the breakdown, win the set pieces, and you're more than halfway to winning the match.
- Work hard off the ball and on the opposition.
- 'Staying alive' so we don't get caught out by the unexpected. Training sessions aren't always structured and organised; some of them are deliberately chaotic and frantic, forcing us not just to think on the hoof but to do so quickly and correctly.
- Being more talkative than they are. Talking creates energy for us and disrupts them. 'Who are you marking?' 'Watch the gap!' 'Nine's stepping out.' All that kind of stuff, but constant and loud. If you're screaming at the top of your voice like a little girl the ref can tell you to shut up, but not if you're saying productive stuff. As Anthrax once sang, bring the noise.

Sunday, 18 June. Team meeting. It's Father's Day back home, and unknown to us the video boys have got everyone's kids to send little clips wishing us a happy day. Anna's first up, and the sight of her nearly finishes me.

Maro Itoje's sitting next to me. 'Whose daughter's that?' he says.

'Mine,' I choke, and I can hardly get the words out. I miss her. I miss her and Rach so much. Sometimes it seems I'm away from home more nights than I'm there. Don't get me wrong, it's a good life, and I know these are opportunities so few people get, but being away from your loved ones is hard no matter who you are. Even seeing Anna's face reminds me of all the things I'm missing, and of all the pressure I'm putting myself under to make sure that this is worth it.

One by one the clips come up: lots of Snapchat filters and 'Happy Father's Day, Daddy' in unison. It's so sweet, and there's scarcely a dry eye in the house. When the clips end, the only sounds are bits of sniffling, with blokes trying desperately not to blub out loud.

'I *need* to get a kid,' Maro says, and the whole room cracks up.

The laughter, however, can't totally disguise a certain amount of discord in the camp. It's to do with the 'geographical six' – Gats's decision to call up six replacements as injury cover for the midweek matches. Every Lions tour needs replacements, as every Lions tour has to deal with injuries severe enough to send original players home.

But those replacements are usually chosen in strict order of merit, and are more often than not blokes who only just missed out in the first place. In 2013, we had to bring in guys like Brad Barritt, Christian Wade, Billy Twelvetrees and Shane Williams. The first three had been close to selection anyway, and though Shane's case was different – he'd retired and happened to be in

Australia at the time – he was also a bona fide rugby legend, a two-time Lions tourist, whose credentials no one could question.

If you get the call-up for the Lions, no matter where in the world you are you drop everything and get on the next flight out, even if that flight ends up being several different flights across multiple time zones. That's the cachet of the Lions. But Gats has chosen to do it differently. Since Wales have just played Tonga in Auckland, and Scotland have just played Australia in Sydney, he's called up Kristian Dacey, Tomas Francis, Cory Hill, Alan Dell, Gareth Davies and Finn Russell, with only the last two probably pretty close to selection originally.

Many of the boys feel that the integrity of the jersey has been compromised. Even one minute in a midweek Lions match is something most Home Nations players get nowhere near. The situation's been made worse by the fact that management didn't initially tell us this was happening. Most of us found out from texts sent by one or more of the six themselves.

So there's a lot of resentment flying around, and inevitably some of it gets taken out on the six new arrivals. They sit at the front of the bus, and abuse is hurled at them from the back, some of it good-natured, or partly so, but some of it with real barbs too.

I go out of my way to sit with the six and try to make them feel welcome, but they know they're not widely wanted and that their presence is unsettling the squad. Cory deals with it well, introducing himself on the bus microphone and saying he won a Twitter competition to be here, and that gets most people back onside, but some of the other six don't seem to know what to say or do. Maybe there's nothing they *can* say or do.

I talk to Gats and let him know the grief this is causing the squad. The irony is that in the end he hardly uses them anyway. Dell and Russell get 15 minutes between them, both as temporary replacements; the four Welsh boys just collect splinters in their arses after two games sitting on the bench. Gats says that he feels unable to use them because of all the controversy, and in any case some of the midweek team make it clear before the start of their games that they'll refuse to be substituted off unless they're injured. They've worked all their careers for this tour, and they don't want to give even a minute on the pitch to someone they feel undeserving of the honour.

The whole affair doesn't disrupt the Test team, so it makes no difference to the series result. But it does disrupt the midweek team, it does add to the pressure I'm putting on myself to be the best captain I can be, and it ends up being a lot of aggro for absolutely no reason whatsoever.

Tuesday, 20 June. Our last midweek match before the Tests, which means it's a pretty good time for the midweek side to notch up their first victory of the tour. It's not just the win that's welcome, but the manner of it too: 34–6 against the Chiefs, and with a real energy and sharpness to boot. That might be enough to put a few of tonight's players in the frame for Saturday, I think; certainly for the bench, maybe even for the starting XV.

Just as we did after the Crusaders match, we all pile into the changing-room and sing our hearts out. Most of the guys who played the Crusaders match sat tonight out and vice versa, which shows how strong the collective spirit is. Whether we're playing or not, we're all in this together.

Wednesday, 21 June. The team for the first Test is announced. I'm on the bench, which given the amount of game time I've been able to have is fair enough and the best I could have hoped for. Pete O'Mahony is captain, which may surprise some people given that Alun Wyn's also in the team, but Pete did a good job as skipper against the Maori All Blacks and is certainly up to the job. Two of last night's team, Liam and Elliot Daly, are in the starting XV for Saturday. It's never too late to put your hand up for selection.

I go over to Pete, shake his hand and tell him I'll give him any help he needs. I know he won't need any, but it's important to make the offer. Everyone goes over to the man who's got his place and shakes his hand, no matter what they might be feeling inside. No one has ever been or ever will be bigger than the Lions.

Geech has always said that the greatest Lion he worked with was Jason Leonard, not for the matches he played but the ones he didn't; for the way he helped Paul Wallace and Tom Smith in South Africa in 1997, despite his own disappointment at not making the Test team.

Just as in 2013, the training session immediately after this announcement is savage, with everyone trying to show either that they deserve their place on Saturday or that they've been unjustly overlooked.

Thursday, 22 June. Just as in 2013, the training session today, once everyone's got yesterday out of their systems, is quick, slick and looking good.

Friday, 23 June. Drico hands out the shirts. He talks about the 1971 vintage, the only Lions ever to have won a tour in New Zealand; in a four-Test series, they won the first and third, lost the second and drew the fourth to take the series 2–1. Whoever heard of the final match of a series being drawn?

That team contained some of the greatest names in rugby history: JPR Williams, Gerald Davies, John Dawes, Mike Gibson, Barry John, Gareth Edwards, Willie John McBride, Mervyn Davies. '1971 is still being talked about like it was yesterday,' Drico says. 'Now it's your turn to make history.'

Saturday, 24 June. Eden Park is lit up like a spaceship. The All Blacks haven't lost here since 1994. Then again, I remember, the Brazil football team hadn't lost at home for something like 40 years when Germany destroyed them 7–1 in the World Cup semi three years ago. Just as I told Sonja McLaughlin after the opening match of the 2013 Six Nations, records are there to be broken.

We come out and line up to face the haka.

The haka. I know it's theatre, I know it's box office, I know that the crowds love it. But I hate it. People say it's a sign of respect. Do me a favour. You're mimicking jabbing me with a spear and cutting my throat. That's not respect. Besides, it never used to be like that. Look at footage of the All Blacks teams in the 1970s. Their body language during the haka was much less confrontational.

Last year, when we came on tour here with Wales, we came to a school that did a haka for us. I was out front as the captain, and there was this big Polynesian kid in front of me giving it all, the staring and eye-rolling and stuff. In the next senior players' meeting, Gats asked us what we were all thinking during that haka. The other boys all said that it was important to respect the local culture, it was part of the experience, and so on.

And I was just thinking, *Please don't ask me*.

'Warby, what do you think?' Gats said.

'Honestly?'

'Of course.'

'I was looking at that big fat kid in front of me, and I was thinking, "Come on, you and me, let's go." I didn't like it. I just wanted to get up and scrap him.'

Gats smiled. 'Exactly. That's exactly what we should be thinking. It's a challenge. You need to eyeball him and tell him with your eyes what you want to do to him.'

I remember that now.

Eyeball them. TJ Perenara prowling as he calls it out.

Eyeball each of them. Kieran Read at the head of the pyramid with Jerome Kaino and Israel Dagg behind him.

Eyeball every last one of them.

The match starts at a furious pace and rarely lets up. We're almost ahead in the first minute when Foxy breaks, Conor's tackled five metres short and Elliot's bundled into the corner by Dagg. A few minutes later, we get a glimpse of what we're up against, when Beauden Barrett scoops the ball up one-handed on the bounce and skips out of Conor's tackle in the same movement.

The All Blacks start to set the tempo, moving the ball fast away from the contact area and working the phases quickly, trying to pull us out of position. Barrett attempts a cross kick to the corner and Anthony (Watson), backpedalling and stretching, does very well to pluck it out of the air.

We try to slow them down, but it's hard to do so without flirting with the law. Barrett kicks one penalty, and then they get another one for not moving away. Once more they're quicker than we are. Aaron Smith taps and passes, it goes through the hands of Barrett and Dagg, and there on the wing is their hooker Codie Taylor, taking it off his own toes and diving in at the corner. Easy to say we were caught napping, but things like that don't happen in isolation. They've been moving us around and taking us to the edge, and that's the result.

We begin to stabilise. Faz has a penalty on the half hour to make it 10–3, only for Barrett to restore the 10-point cushion three minutes later. We need something before half-time, something that won't just get us closer on the scoreboard but will also show the All Blacks and the crowd that we can play some rugby just the way they can.

Five minutes before the break, we get it.

Anthony fields an Aaron Cruden box kick in our 22 and passes infield to Liam. Read's hammering up the middle towards Liam, but rather than kick, Liam chooses to be matador to Read's bull, dropping his shoulder and stepping him so expertly that Read looks exasperatedly towards the heavens as his momentum takes him forward into thin air.

Liam running flatstick across the 22, looking for the space. Sonny Bill coming across before Ben blocks his run, subtly but perfectly. Cruden trying to close Liam down, but Liam's too quick and now he has the angle to head upfield.

Liam running in open space with red and black shirts scrambling in his wake. The crowd rising, sensing something. Liam running with his head up and looking all around him, seeing where the support and the danger is. Liam up to halfway. Liam taking Dagg's tackle and feeding Foxy. Foxy onto Elliot. Elliot adjusting his line, in then out, fixing Anton Leinert-Brown. Elliot back inside to Foxy. Foxy turning Barrett left then right. Barrett getting to Foxy. Foxy spinning himself in the tackle to feed Sean two metres from the line, and over Sean goes with Smith and Dagg clinging onto him.

Try. What a try. The Lions can't play rugby? Watch that and weep.

It's 13–8 to the All Blacks at half-time.

'It's a man test,' says Andy Farrell. 'Are we ready for it?'

We start the second half as though we are, that's for sure. Twice Liam and Anthony combine to beat men. They look dangerous, not just with their own lines but in the way they're opening the doors to our other runners. But we can't break through, and there's no team better than the All Blacks in soaking up pressure and then hitting you on the counter.

With 53 minutes gone, I come on for Pete. I've got half an hour to help win the game and ensure I start the second Test, and each of those feeds off the other.

A minute after my arrival, Read shows why the All Blacks value him so much. The ball comes loose on the floor, and even though he hasn't played for six weeks he's first there, scooping a pass off the floor purely through the power in his fingers. He doesn't have a backlift with his hand, let alone his arm. Just flicks it up with his fingers, and down the line it goes for Ioane to slide in at the corner.

Barrett converts, and then nails a penalty on the hour to make it 23–8. We're more than two converted tries behind now, so we have to chase the game, even if that means leaving ourselves open. With just over ten minutes to go we try to work it up the right side, but it comes loose in traffic. Perenara hoists the kick, Liam – usually so secure under the high ball that he's nicknamed 'the Bomb Defuser' – drops it, the bounce falls kindly for Ioane, and he scorches Elliot on the outside. With the conversion, that's 30–8 and game more or less over.

I keep competing like crazy at the breakdown, just to try and slow things down and provide some damage control. It's a shit job, putting your head in there time after time, but I love doing it. The adrenaline masks the pain. The pain's always there now.

We pressure them hard at the end, desperate to come away with something to take into next week. Faz drills a penalty to the corner and we win the lineout. The clock's gone red now. Rhys Webb darts and is caught. Foxy smashes through a couple of tackles and sets up the ruck. Again Rhys darts, this time throwing a dummy round the fringes, and he's through for a try: 30–15.

The All Blacks were the better team and good value for the win, there's no doubt about that. They were also the first team we've played on tour who got the better of us physically, which was one of the main reasons they won.

'Our energy wasn't good enough,' Andy says. 'We were our own worst enemies. The amount of times we had the All Blacks exactly where we wanted them and then let them out far too easily with a penalty, an offside, a dropped ball, whatever – we didn't manage our energy well enough and the physicality went backwards on the back of that.'

He's right. But four things stand out for me. First, the margin of victory flattered them. They might have been a score better, but not two scores plus better. Second, we scored two tries to their three, and at least one of theirs was sloppy defending on our part and a lucky bounce on theirs. Third, we're not going to lose the physical battle again. And finally, we're still improving.

This series isn't over yet, not by a long chalk.

Sunday, 25 June. I feel battered, absolutely battered, even though I played less than half an hour. I'm used to the pain, but this is different. I'm operating some way off my maximum capacity, and sometimes I feel like I'm just hanging on. I'm undercooked, I haven't got time to get back to anything like full fitness, and I feel that I might snap at any moment.

Monday, 26 June. I have to hide it all. I have to be in the team, and we have to win. That's all there is to it. Park the doubts, shelve the pain. Grit my teeth and push on through. Whatever it takes. Whatever it takes.

Tuesday, 27 June. The midweek team's last match, against the Hurricanes. We're 16 points up at half-time, but somehow let the Hurricanes back in to snatch a 31–31 draw. It's a frantic, thrilling match, which the crowd love, and though we really should have won it, at least we didn't lose.

Now there are only two matches left, the second and third Tests, and we have to win them both.

Wednesday, 28 June. I'm as fit as I'm going to be. If I'm not in the starting XV tomorrow, it'll be because the coaches don't think I'm good enough. Gats dropped Drico four years ago. He'd drop me in a heartbeat too, which is why he's such a good coach. No sentiment, not when it matters.

I could go and ask to sit in on the selection meeting. He's always said I'm welcome at them. But I've never done that before and I can't start now, no matter how desperate I am to find out whether I'm in.

Thursday, 29 June. I almost cry when he reads my name out in the team meeting. I'm back in the starting XV, as skipper. Pete's dropped altogether, with the coaches preferring CJ's versatility on the bench. It's a tough call for Pete – from captain one week to spectator the next – but it just shows how high our standards are and how intense the competition for places is.

I tell the press conference that this is the biggest challenge of my career, which it is. It's the biggest challenge of all our careers, from Gats downwards. 'We know it's all or nothing now. When you've been physically outplayed, which we were, that does hurt you as a playing group. In rugby it's very much a case of 99 times out of 100 the more physical team wins. Being physical doesn't mean beating up people. It means your scrum is dominant, your lineout maul is dominant and your breakdown is dominant. We all accept last weekend was probably the first game on tour we were beaten in the battle at the breakdown from a physicality point of view. That's just going to fuel the fire.'

I'm not just saying these things. I truly believe them, and myself. That's what helps make people believe me too. But the level of anticipation for this match is scaring me. Even at the press conference, I could feel it; the reporters, hard-bitten at the best of times and usually by now knackered from weeks on the road, are really up for it. Am I up for it? Am I up to it? Is my body going to let me down again?

Two in the morning.

Can't sleep. The witching hour, when the darkness comes flooding in; thoughts tumbling and cascading over each other like a Snowdonia river in full spate. The darkness comes flooding in, and it's all I can do to stop it drowning me.

I get out of bed. Shards of pain as my feet touch the floor. I push myself slowly upright, gritting my teeth as the aches flare and settle.

Sam Warburton shouldn't be captain.

Sam Warburton shouldn't be playing.

Sam Warburton's past it.

I take one step, gingerly, then another, and another. Walking – hobbling, more like – across the carpet over to the window. I pull back the curtains and look out.

Below me is the Wellington waterfront. It's quiet and empty now, but earlier this evening it was packed, as it will be later tonight, and tomorrow night, and Saturday night too. Many of these people will be wearing red rugby shirts, and will have saved up for years to come all the way across the world just to watch us play.

I want to be one of those fans, drinking and singing their hearts out, with no problem more pressing than who gets the next round in. Instead, I'm here, torturing myself with questions to which I have no answer. *Why? Why am I doing this to myself? Why am I putting myself through all this pain, all this pressure, when I could be doing something – anything – else? Why am I in a job which right now I detest?*

Round and round and round. Body, mind and heart. Physical stress, mental stress and emotional stress, all working on and off each other. I feel as though I'm in a submarine going deeper and deeper, springing leaks as the hull creaks and flexes, and soon I'll come to the point of no return, the moment when the pressure gets too much and crushes me like a tin can.

A submarine. A volcano. All this pain bubbling up inside me, and if I don't deal with it, it's going to explode and consume me in all its molten fury.

I need to talk to someone. There are several people I could call, but there's only one person I know will really understand. I dial her number.

'Sam?' Her voice is full of concern. It's lunchtime back home in Cardiff. She knows what time it is where I am, and that I wouldn't be phoning for no reason.

'I've had enough, Mum.'

Friday, 30 June. Not much sleep, but feeling a bit better having spoken to Mum.

We have our captain's run at the Jerry Collins Stadium in Porirua. I would love to have played against Collins – he retired before I began my international career – and I've heard all about him: a huge guy known as 'the Terminator' for the ferocity of his tackling, but off the pitch a lovely man who'd go into bars and chat to fans, who once played for Barnstaple seconds while on holiday in Devon just because he fancied a game (and who then asked Barnstaple if he could wear their socks when he turned out for the Barbarians), and who was killed two years ago in a car crash at the age of only 34. His last act was to throw himself over his baby daughter and save her life.

It's some perspective, a reminder of something that I badly need to remember right now: no matter how important tomorrow is, it's still just a game.

Saturday, 1 July. The second Test of three is always huge, as one team's fighting to stay in the series. Four years ago it was Australia; now it's us. There's a purity to that equation. Game on or game over, make or break, win or bust.

'We're hurting more than them,' Graham Rowntree, the Lions assistant coach, says. 'Use that energy. They're in for a f***ing long night.'

I gather the boys round me. 'Sometimes it comes down to this.' I beat my fist against my heart. 'Who's the bravest? Who wants it more? Who's the most hungry? Tonight it's us.'

It's sheeting it down at the Westpac, but the fans don't care. They're a sea of red, singing and dancing, every one of them soaked to the skin, but the atmosphere is still so passionate that you can almost touch it.

And that passion, that energy, comes from within us too. We have to dredge the depths of our souls to make this the game of our lives, of all our lives. This is a level above almost anything else in sport.

The most important 80 minutes of my career. Here we go.

The All Blacks lay out their tactics right from the start: Smith makes two box kicks in the first 90 seconds, trying to unsettle our back three. It's not just wet, but windy too, and when Liam chases his own high kick, both he and Dagg miss it as it drops.

Conor and Elliot work it up the short side. Jérôme Garcès pings the All Blacks for not rolling away. I win the lineout and Tadhg Furlong makes the hard yards, dragging Kaino with him. Those big physical sessions we had on Tuesday and Thursday have really paid off. We're not letting ourselves be outmuscled again.

Johnny feints to send Sonny Bill the wrong way. Foxy flips a pass to Alun Wyn out of the back of his hand. The first 10 minutes are all ours; they've hardly been in our half, and we're playing all the rugby.

Eleven minutes gone, and they get down our end for pretty much the first time. Barrett has a penalty, but it hits the upright and bounces back into play. A few minutes later, Read knocks on. Last week, Barrett didn't miss a kick and Read was immaculate. Not today. Small margins, but small margins win big games.

We front up to the All Blacks at a maul. Not one step back, not from any of us. But Mako's penalised for going down at the scrum, and this time Barrett does nail the kick. We're level within a few minutes, and it's from something Gats flagged to Garcès earlier in the week: the All Blacks runners being ahead of Smith when he box-kicks.

The rain is hammering down – proper monsoon conditions.

With 24 minutes gone, the game changes irrevocably. Toby catches a Sonny Bill kick and offloads to Anthony. It's not the greatest offload, and by the time Anthony's got it and looped round there are two men on him. Waisake Naholo is first to get him, and as he makes the tackle Sonny Bill drops his arms and shoulder-charges Anthony straight in the face.

The crowd gasp. Garcès blows his whistle. Johnny and Faz come sprinting towards the ruck, screaming in protest. Anthony is down on his knees, groggy from the hit.

'Warby!' Faz shouts. 'Speak to the ref! Shoulder to head's a straight red!'

I look at Garcès. He's already talking to the TMO, so I know they're going to have a look. That's all I need to know. No point spending my chips on this one. If the hit's as bad as it looked, Garcès will see that and he'll make the right decision. If it's not, no amount of me getting in his face will make a difference.

I turn back to Faz. 'Mate, leave it. They're taking a look.'

The replay comes up on the big screen. It's every bit as bad as it first looked, maybe worse. You can see the fear in Anthony's eyes in the last half-second before the impact, when he knows what's coming and tries to duck his face away. Every time the hit is shown and Anthony's head snaps back the crowd wince, and the Lions fans are booing and whistling, because it looks more and more like a straight red each time.

No referee has ever sent an All Black off in a Test on New Zealand soil.

I'd better have got this right.

Garcès walks over to Sonny Bill. He has the red card in his hand. 'I have no choice,' he says. 'Direct shoulder to the head.

I need to protect the player. It's direct. The contact is direct.' He holds the card high, and off Sonny Bill goes.

I bring all the boys in and tell them that this is our chance. I remember doing an event at Celtic Manor with Gareth Edwards, and he was talking about pressing home an advantage. 'When you've got your foot on your opponent's throat,' he said – and you could almost see him transforming back to the player he'd been even as he said this – 'when you've got your foot on your opponent's throat, you keep it there.'

We need to keep our foot on their throat now. We're a man up with 55 minutes still left to play. We'll never have a better chance than this. If we don't take it then we don't deserve to win in the first place.

Sean and I drive forward, but we snatch at the ball and it goes down. There's a thin line between pressing home an advantage and trying too hard, and we're veering towards the latter. In conditions like this you have to let things come to you, you have to make things happen without forcing them. Easier said than done.

Conor tackles Barrett and is pinged for not rolling away. Barrett fades the kick nicely from right to left. The All Blacks are ahead again. They don't seem fazed by being a man down; in fact, they seem to be embracing it as a challenge.

Faz brings it back to 6–6. Mako is caught on his knee at a ruck, and that's 9–6. With the hooter already gone for the end of the half, we get a penalty and try to work the advantage. Conor, thinking fast, cross kicks for Toby to jump with Ioane. The ball goes loose and Anthony slides in to try to grab it, but he just can't make it. No matter. It was a free play, so back we go for the penalty; and that's 9–9 at half-time.

In the changing-room, thinking our way through the game. Our line speed is good in midfield and we're squeezing them well round the fringes, making a mess of their ball, picking their runners off well, making them play behind the gainline. Last week they won the breakdown; today it's ours. We're giving Smith at 9 much less time than before, forcing him to hurry his kicks and passes. Keep doing all this and we'll win.

Two minutes into the second half, Barrett gets a very kickable penalty. For the second time tonight, he misses. His radar's off. We have to use that.

Four minutes later, Conor goes high on Leinert-Brown, and this time Barrett makes no mistake: 12–9. Now it's all them, Dagg slicing through, Barrett skewing a grubber kick that would have put Read clean through for a try if he'd got it right. Ninety per cent of the first ten minutes has been played in our half.

Mako comes in late on Barrett. No, he tells Garcès, I didn't change my line. I shepherd him away before he pisses Garcès off even more. Barrett sneaks his kick inside the left-hand post, and we're six points down. On 55 minutes Mako is pinged again, this time for clearing Barrett out at a ruck with his right forearm cocked, and now Garcès has had enough. He sends Mako to the bin, and Barrett kicks the penalty: 18–9.

Yes, they're putting us under pressure, but that's three unnecessary penalties given away, nine needless points conceded, and now we've lost our one-man advantage for 10 minutes. The All Blacks don't even need to try and win this. We're losing it all by ourselves.

On 59 minutes, Sean tackles Naholo so hard that Naholo has to go off. The All Blacks rejig their shape quickly and expertly: Cruden on at 10, Barrett shifting to 15 and Dagg out to 14.

This is our chance. We haven't used the extra man at all well, but now we're down to 14 on 14 we have to take the initiative, and that starts by finding where the mismatches are and using them. There's a mismatch now.

Johnny and Faz run at their midfield, holding the defence while they distribute. Out it comes to Liam, who feeds Toby on the left wing. Dagg comes to tackle, but he's not as big or solid as Naholo. Toby bounces him off and dives in at the corner as Retallick tries to cover.

I'm first to Toby, hugging him and screaming in his ear. The Lions fans are going potty in the stands. The only person who doesn't seem that bothered is Toby himself, but then nothing seems to get to him.

If you want to know why Toby's such a special player, it's all there in that try. Lots of players would have had the strength to bounce Dagg off, and lots of players would have had the speed and skill to dive in at the corner before the cover hit came in, but very few players would have had both. Toby does.

Faz shanks the conversion badly, so it stays 18–14. But we're still in this. We're still very much in this.

A wall of sound from the stands. *Liiiions! Liiiions! Liiiions!*

Still the All Blacks come. Ngani Laumape drives forward and takes Johnny back yards as he clings on. Cruden overcooks a grubber for Read, but they have the penalty anyway, and the gap's back to seven points.

Thirteen minutes left. Johnny feeds Jamie George, who's still full of running – in fact, he'll play the whole 80, almost unheard of for a hooker at this level. Jamie's brought down, and from the ruck Conor snipes and scores. Perenara moans that Faz was holding his ankle, stopping him from getting to Johnny, but Garcès isn't having any of it. Faz converts: 21–21. Twelve minutes left.

Time to look each other in the eye. Time to believe.

A draw is not enough. A draw means we can't win the series, we can only square it. New Zealand with 47 straight wins at home. The weight of all those wins pressing down on both sides. Play the game in front of you, nothing else.

A scrum on halfway. Conor uses the ball to shield his mouth as he checks the calls with Johnny. These two know each other so well, and that's vital in situations like this: the clutch, the quick, the moment where you either have it or you don't.

Four minutes left. Sinks comes hard off 9, but the pass is a touch high and he needs to jump to take it. At the exact moment he's in the air, Charlie Faumuina makes the tackle. Garcès blows immediately.

Penalty.

The All Blacks are furious. Faumuina was committed to the tackle before Sinks jumped, there was clearly no attempt to injure him, and Faumuina's only alternative was to pull out and wave Sinks through.

'I didn't know he'd jump,' Faumuina says.

'So next time I jump and they tackle me, is that OK?' Read adds.

It's a harsh penalty, perhaps, but it's also a correct one according to the letter of the law, and Garcès doesn't have much choice other than to give it. Sinks is chopsing off at a few of the All Blacks who are giving him grief. Jamie, Sean and Foxy pull him away before Garcès can change his mind.

The kick is 33 metres out. Faz has got four out of five so far. He's already walking towards the spot, head down.

'Three?' I say as he passes me.

He raises his head and looks at me as though it's the stupidest question he's ever heard.

He takes the tee and sets it down. The routine, always the routine. Putting the valve of the ball at the front, aiming down the centreline of the posts, so that the ball's pointing in the direction he needs to kick it. Taking his steps back. Into his stance. Looking down at the ball and up at the posts, two, three, four times; drawing a line in his head from the ball to a spot far beyond the posts. Drawing that line. Drawing that line.

The first step. The way he holds his body back and upright just for a moment before taking the last few strides. The contact, boot on ball.

I never, not for a nanosecond, think he's going to miss.

There are 2 minutes and 55 seconds left when the ball goes over. We're ahead for the first time this series, and now we have to hold out, to weather the storm – and we all know the storm's coming. It's the All Blacks. They never go down without making you give all you've got.

Ardie Savea takes it off the restart. He goes down in the tackle but he's not held. He gets up and makes 20 metres with men hanging off him. The All Blacks work it left but drop it. Foxy kicks it on, Barrett collects and hands Faz off. Dagg takes it into contact.

Stay onside. No penalties. Whatever you do, no penalties. Soak it up and keep soaking. Bend, but don't break.

Cruden kicks crossfield. Laumape can't get there. Foxy shepherds it into touch.

Our lineout. I'm at the front, and I have this sudden thought: *use the flash call.* The flash call overrides a normal call, and you can use it when you know you're unmarked. They haven't got anyone on me.

Step out of the calling process and react to what you see. Take it on yourself. You're a big man. Back yourself.

Flash call. Flash call.

It's risky. I might not make myself heard, or the boys may be too busy listening for the normal call. But Jamie and Sean hear all right, and as long as the thrower and lifter are on the same page as you then you're in business.

I jump and claim it. Conor kicks clear, and there's a wall of red shirts chasing it up the field. Almost the whole match gone, when the boys should be out on their feet, and we're outrunning New Zealand as though we're possessed.

This is what it takes: to want it just that little bit more, to find the moment when you have the will to do what the other team won't.

One minute left.

The ball comes loose. Conor volleys it clear. Anywhere will do as long as it's upfield, but in fact it's perfect, rolling into touch in their 22. They take a quick lineout to Barrett, who tries a chip over the top. It's the wrong decision, and that's because he's rattled. Games have gone their way so often, so when their key decision-makers make mistakes, that's when you know you're into them.

Sean collects it and takes it up. He takes men, and metres, and time.

Thirty seconds.

Ruck.

Twenty.

I have it. Wyatt Crockett makes the tackle and I go to ground.

Ten.

The Lions fans start counting down.

Courtney Lawes takes it into contact with Jamie on his shoulder.

The hooter goes. Time up. Next time the ball goes dead, the match is over.

Conor takes it from the base of the ruck and boots it into the crowd.

Graham Simmons from Sky Sports grabs me for an on-pitch interview.

'Is this tell your grandchildren time?' he asks.

I get that it's a hell of an achievement, being the first team to beat New Zealand on their own turf in 48 matches, and I get that he's only looking for a reaction, but this is what I mean by being happy to win just one match. One match is only one match. It's not enough.

'It's only half a job done,' I reply. 'I'll be happy next week when we bring the Test series home. We've got to win the Test series. It's great that we've got it to one-all. We wanted to take it to Eden Park. But we've still got plenty to work on. We gave away too many penalties in the second half, and we've got to remember it was against 14 men.'

I'm happy, don't get me wrong. But I'm happy only that we've kept the series alive. If we don't win next week, then all this will have been for nothing.

Most of the boys are celebrating. There's a bit of afters between Sinks and Perenara. I help to break it up. For such a ferociously competitive series it's been played in a pretty good spirit so far, and I want to keep it that way.

We sing 'Fields of Athenry' in the dressing-room afterwards, and it feels as good as it sounds. When the singing dies down, Faz speaks. 'Let's keep it low key,' he says. 'This is what we'll get used to, as we're doing it next week as well.'

I couldn't have said it better myself.

Read is gracious in defeat, saying that we were the better side and that they won't use the red card as an excuse for their defeat. Sam Cane's also humble and says nice things, but it's his three-word reply to a question about the decider next week that stays with me.

'Game on, mate.'

A few of the guys go out on the town. I don't even think of doing so. Why should I? I've come here to win the series, nothing less. All this win has done is ensured we have the chance to do so.

It's like an Olympic athlete winning a semi-final; a win that means nothing in itself other than keeping him in the hunt for the ultimate prize. In fact, I remember speaking to Darren Campbell, who won gold in the 4x100 metre relay in the 2004 Olympics, about this.

'Would you have drunk a few beers a week before your Olympic final?' I asked.

'Of course not,' he said.

Well, this – the third Test against the All Blacks – is our Olympic final.

Sunday, 2 July. Bobby shows us the GPS figures from yesterday.

'Look at the graphs here,' he says, pointing to an upwards curve on the right-hand side. 'You know what that means? That in the last 20 minutes, when the intensity always falls off because guys are tired, your KPIs actually went up.'

I think of the red wave near the end, all of us racing past the All Blacks to get to the lineout first.

'That *never* happens,' Bobby continues. 'Even when you use all the bench, the cumulative numbers always go down in the last quarter. This is the first time I've ever seen this, and I've been doing this gig a long time.'

That's the kind of commitment to the cause we needed to win against the best team in the world; and that, and more, is what we'll need to win against them twice in a row. No All Black takes losing well, and nor should they. It's why they're the best in the world. As one journalist writes: 'There is hurt pride, and then there is the savage, iron will of an All Black looking to atone for his sins.' We all know which one we'll be up against on Saturday.

Monday, 3 July. We have a couple of days off in central Otago, where the boys can go jetskiing or bungee jumping. It's the same kind of break we had in Noosa after the second Test four years ago, and that did us a world of good.

We don't want to get so wound up and keen to crack on that we peak too soon. 'It's mental refreshment, so we don't play our game too early,' Bobby says. The final Test is on Saturday. If we're ready to play it by Thursday, that's no good. Hence the break.

Wednesday, 5 July. Gats names an unchanged 23, which is no small testament to the work of the physios in keeping us fit at the end of a savage tour. It's the first time in 24 years that the same Lions XV has played two consecutive Tests.

If anything shows you how hard the Lions is, it's this. The two titans of the 2013 tour were Pence and George. They didn't get a Test between them in 2017. Only six of us – Foxy, Johnny, Alun Wyn, Sean, Toby and me – started Tests in both tours.

The list of those who've started Tests in three tours in the professional era is even shorter: Drico, Paulie, Alun Wyn and Neil Back.

There's a backlash headed our way, and the Irish boys in the squad know that better than anyone. Ireland beat the All Blacks in Chicago last November, but two weeks later in Dublin they couldn't live with the fury of the All Blacks' revenge. 'I remember coming off the pitch and being absolutely shattered,' Tadhg says. 'I was sore for days after it. It was one of the most brutal Test matches I've played.'

Thursday, 6 July. The New Zealand press are scared. I can tell that by the questions their journalists are asking at the press conference. Like Mako said: you *definitely* know who we are now.

In one way, the pressure's off. Whatever happens on Saturday, this tour will have been a success commercially and in terms of fan involvement. We no longer have to worry about letting people down or betraying the very concept of the Lions. We know we've done the Lions proud.

But as a player, that's not enough. How many of us will ever be in this position again, with the prospect of a Lions series win against the All Blacks? Maro, maybe. Perhaps Tadhg. No one else. This is our one chance, our one shot at that. This is our date with destiny.

Friday, 7 July. John Spencer, the tour manager, tells us that his phone's been pinging with texts from the guys who were on the 1971 tour with him. 'All of them have been saying: "Get this monkey off our backs. We don't want to die with the record around our necks."'

71/17: it has a nice symmetry.

The locals are talking up the Eden Park record something rotten. You might have won last week, the message goes, but you won't win here, not at a ground where no visiting side has won in the professional era. But I don't buy all this Fortress Eden Park stuff. Grounds are strips of grass, nothing more. What matters is not where you are; what matters is turning your plans into reality.

One last spin of the roulette wheel. Red or black?

Saturday, 8 July. 'It's about having emotional control,' Gats says. 'You want to take it to the edge, but you don't want to go over the top.' In other words: fire in the soul, ice in the veins.

Andy stands up and looks at us. 'I believe today you'll become the best team in the world,' he says.

Putting on the strapping like armour. I've done this hundreds of times in my career, and as I wind it tight now I have a sudden feeling.

This is my last game.

I've never thought beyond the next 80 minutes, but this feels different. *This is my last game. This is the last time I'll ever do this.*

It's every player's dream to go out not just on their own terms but right at the top. The only other man to captain the Lions twice was Martin Johnson, and his last international was the 2003 World Cup Final. Not a bad way to go out. For my last game to be the series clincher against the All Blacks – well, that would be right up there. Eighty minutes of pain for glory that would last a lifetime.

I pull the boys in. The red Lions jerseys seem to glow, lit by fires from within.

'Let's pass this jersey on to the next generation,' I tell them.

No one owns a Lions jersey. You just carry it for a few weeks, try to add to it and pass it on. It's not the jersey you put on that matters; it's the one you take off.

Empty the tank, Gats said. *We'll take the shirt off for you at the end if need be.*

We go out into the corridor. All the midweek boys and the support staff are there, slapping our backs as we pass. I pick up BIL, our Lions mascot.

Out of the tunnel as if coming up for air. *Liiiions! Liiiions! Liiiions!* A depth and growl to the chants, knowing how close we are to history, knowing what an inestimable privilege it would be to say you were there when it happened. I drop BIL on the ground the moment my boots go over the whitewash.

Take it in. Take it all in. This is the last time you'll ever play.

The All Blacks set themselves for the haka. I'm watching them, but for once I'm not thinking how much I hate it. I'm thinking of everything that's brought me here, all the hundreds and thousands of tiny things which have led to this moment: me, Sam Warburton, captaining the Lions at 1–1 against New Zealand.

It's fitting that my last game will be in a Lions shirt, because for me this has always been the ultimate. Geech put it very well once. 'That badge represents four countries, but it also represents you. You should be carrying that badge for people who have put you in that position. It might be a schoolmaster, mother, father, brother, sister, wife, girlfriend. Whatever's special to you, the people who have brought you to this place, that's who you should be wearing it for. That's who you should be playing for. Because in the end they're the ones who matter. They matter to you. And if it matters to you, it will matter to all of us. And if it matters to us, we will win. Go out, enjoy it, but play for everything that's in the badge. For you personally, for all of us collectively.'

Perenara starts the call and response for the haka.

Taringa whakarongo!

Kia rite! Kia rite! Kia mau!

Hi!

Playing with the Under-14s at Whitchurch, on a pitch exactly the same size and shape as this. Realising that I might be quite good. Great team, great bunch of blokes. The WhatsApp group we're all part of now, bonded by those memories. The match so long ago that the tape we have of it is VCR rather than DVD.

Kia whakawhenua au i ahau!

Hi, aue! Hi!

Blood and thunder against the Irish in Wellington. Our red line spread across the pitch, soaking up their pressure, making them punch themselves out. Foxy scoring and their heads going down, and from the stands the fans singing 'Delilah' over and over.

Ko Aotearoa, e ngunguru nei!

Hi, au! Au! Aue, ha! Hi!

The trophy lift in the darkness after taking England's Grand Slam away from them at the Millennium. Punching the air in triumph at the crowd, and three tiers of people punching the air in unison back at me. Rock-star time.

Ko kapa o pango, e ngunguru nei!

Hi, au! Au! Aue, ha! Hi!

Geech handing me my first Lions Test jersey. Laying that jersey out on my bed, the number 7 looking up at me, just as it had done on the replica I'd worn when I was 15.

I ahaha!

Ka tu te ihi-ihi

Ka tu te wanawana

Ki runga i te rangi, e tu iho nei, tu iho nei, hi!

Coming on against Italy and hearing the crowd roar my name. Their appreciation that I turned down Toulon to stay in Wales and sign the central contract. The tears in my eyes as I run across the pitch to the lineout.

Ponga ra!

Kapa o pango! Aue, hi!

My 100th game for the Blues on Boxing Day. The whole family there; all the people I love most gathered in a place that's very special to me. Baby Anna seeing her dad playing for the first time.

Ponga ra!

Kapa o pango! Aue, hi!

Ha!

The texts my Dad sends me before every match, always ending with the same four words in block capitals: REFUSE TO BE DENIED.

REFUSE TO BE DENIED. The dream I had. The pledge I made.

The haka ends. I count to five before moving, like we all do; we've agreed that beforehand, that we'll wait a few moments and let the All Blacks turn away first. Flames fire into the sky.

We line up for the kick-off. Johnny bounces the ball on the ground. Romain Poite checks with both sides that we're ready. I've never felt more ready. It's almost as though this is a funnel, with everything in my life poured into the top and narrowed down to this match and this match alone.

Poite whistles. I watch the ball fall from Johnny's hands as he drop-kicks.

Showtime.

Less than 90 seconds gone when Beauden Barrett takes it into contact and I rip it from him. No, says Poite, that's an illegal turnover. It wasn't. I know it wasn't. It was a perfectly good steal. I'm on form, so that's good to know.

Barrett misses the penalty. Laumape chips, Elliot gathers and is caught. Conor clears from the ruck, but back they come again from a free-kick. Smith taps and goes, Beauden Barrett on to his brother Jordie, out to Julian Savea with the line beckoning ... and Savea knocks on when he'd have been in for the score.

Five minutes gone, and we've barely been in their half.

I make a second steal, this time off Retallick. We have a chance to break, but Faz knocks on. Just like they did on this ground a fortnight ago, the All Blacks are trying to play at a pace too high for us, trying to nullify our physicality by constantly moving the ball away. We have to leach the sting from them and slow it down.

Nine minutes gone. Maro steals, but Faz puts it out on the full. We get it back and start to make inroads. Johnny makes a half-break, then Maro, then Elliot. Give it to the heavy boys. Tadhg and Jamie take it up to within five metres. Fifteen phases and counting, and now Conor spins it wide and we have an overlap out on the right, Liam and Anthony doubling up on their last man. Get it through the hands and we'll score. Faz throws the pass ...

... and Jordie Barrett plucks it out of the air for the intercept.

Suddenly we're all chasing back. Liam runs Barrett down, but he pops it out of the tackle to Laumape who pins his ears back and goes for the corner. Foxy's after him. Laumape's quick, but Foxy's quicker. Foxy runs him down and catches him 15 metres out. The ball comes loose to Anthony, who collects it and Savea at the same time, and in the blink of an eye we've gone from being five metres out from their line to five metres out from ours. Conor clears.

That's three uncharacteristic mistakes from Faz with barely ten minutes gone, more than he's made in the first two Tests put together. It happens, sometimes. And if there's anyone with the mental strength to shrug off this kind of thing, it's Faz.

The All Blacks are still laying siege to our line. I try to get my hands on the ball, but there are too many bodies in the way.

Out it comes to Beauden Barrett, who cross kicks for his brother in the corner. Jordie gets up above Elliot and palms it down for Laumape to scoot in before Foxy, still exhausted from his earlier chase, can get to him. Once more they've scored first.

Now we start to get some kind of footing. Foxy puts a grubber through and Elliot bundles Beauden Barrett into touch. This is fast, furious and unrelenting.

Penalty to us with exactly a quarter of the match gone. Faz, ice cool from the tee as always, makes it 7–3.

Again Beauden Barrett puts up a cross kick, this time for Savea. Savea beats Faz and runs over Liam, but Faz tracks back to make the tackle second time round. There's another black wave breaking over us, but Cane knocks on and Toby gathers, drops and gathers again.

Our scrum, right on our line. The ball's held between the two front rows, right in the tunnel. Pressure and force and muscle for tiny gains. The All Blacks wheel and disrupt, getting a secondary shunt on. Smith pops it up to Beauden Barrett, who knocks on with Toby covering.

It's our pressure that's making them make mistakes – the more opportunities they squander, the tighter they'll get and the more likely they are to snatch at the next chance too – but we can't keep playing this rope-a-dope for ever.

The All Blacks take the next scrum down and Johnny clears, but he doesn't find touch and back they come again. Smith box-kicks, Liam spills and now the All Blacks are over the gainline again and we're going backwards. It's been a long, long time since we were anywhere near their posts. *Red line in D. Red line in D.* Laumape knocks on when he's almost through and finally Conor gives us some breathing space when he clears to halfway.

If the All Blacks had held on to all their passes, they'd be out of sight.

Half an hour gone. Foxy clatters Beauden Barrett and I jackal long enough to get the penalty. Faz nails it and we're within a point of them, though I'm not quite sure how. We'll have done well if we can get to half-time like this.

We can't. Five minutes before the break, they work it through the hands off a lineout and a lovely floated pass sends Jordie Barrett in for a try on debut.

It's 12–6 at the break. Could have been worse. Should have been worse.

Johnny speaks up in the changing-room. 'The moment we have them on the track, we let them off the hook. It's there for the f***ing taking if we want it.'

Beauden Barrett's kick-off to start the second half doesn't go 10 metres; the kind of mistake a club player shouldn't make, let alone the best 10 in the world. That's pressure for you. Foxy takes it on and Read obstructs Liam. Our penalty, just inside our half. Kick to the 22 and work the lineout?

'I'll have a go,' Elliot says.

He's got a monster kick on him, and in training he puts them over from this kind of distance for fun. But a 55-metre kick six points down in the biggest match of your life is a whole different ask to the practice pitch.

He looks confident. And if a kicker's confident, then trust him.

Elliot doesn't have an elaborate routine, take a particularly long run-up or seem to connect any harder than any other kicker, but bloody hell he gives this one a thump. It's high enough and straight enough, and it gets over with a yard or two to spare. What a kick. What a start to the second half.

The All Blacks work a maul and then send Jordie Barrett and Savea down the left. Liam steps up smartly on Barrett, forcing him to hurry the pass and make it forward. They're playing wide much better than we are, but they're also making twice as many handling errors as we are, doing what we did for long parts of the Wellington Test, trying to force the game rather than let it come.

Half an hour left. Alun Wyn's clattered by Kaino and Whitelock together: Kaino's stiff-arm to the jaw, knocking Alun Wyn unconscious for a moment or two, his head going back and his eyes closing. Ten minutes in the bin for Kaino.

This third quarter is where we almost let it slip last time. We can't afford to do the same thing tonight, and we don't. Now three-quarters of the possession is ours. Anthony and Liam work it down the right again. Foxy scythes down Jordie Barrett. Retallick comes in high on Courtney and Liam's in Retallick's face, size difference be damned. Our penalty, and Faz nails it.

Twenty minutes to go: 12–12 in the match, 1–1 in the series. Two teams who just can't be separated.

It's there for the taking if we want it.

I fly out of the line and into Crockett, making him spill. So close to offside, but we can't afford to give anything away now. Foxy and Elliot go up the left-hand side. Both sides are going for it with all they've got now, no quarter asked, no holds barred. Empty the tank.

Fifteen minutes left. I go low to tackle Read and his knee smacks into my head. I get back up and into line – *unless you're unconscious or you've snapped your femur you get back in D –* but my head's thumping and I don't know what's north or south. At the next break, Poite tells me to go off for an HIA. I jog off the pitch as quick as I can. Every second counts.

The medics take me to a room below the stadium and run through the HIA protocols.

'What venue are we at today?'

'Eden Park.'

A cheer from the crowd, filtering muffled through the walls.

'Which half is it now?'

'Second.'

No crescendo, so not the excitement of the few seconds before a try.

'Who scored last in this match?'

'We did.'

It sounded loud enough to have been them and not us.

'What team did you play last week?'

'The All Blacks.'

Three points to them, if I had to guess.

'Did your team win the last game?'

'Yes.'

It's 15–12. We can still do this.

'OK. I'm going to read out five words, and I want you to repeat them back to me. Do you understand?'

'Yes.'

I'm captain. I have to get back on now.

'Baby. Monkey. Perfume. Sunset. Iron.'

'Baby. Monkey. Perfume. Sunset. Iron.'

We've got a lock filling in for me at six, and that's not good.

'Now I'm going to read out number strings, and I want you to repeat them back to me in reverse order. Four, three, nine.'

'Nine, three, four.'

What if they make a mistake I'd never have made and that loses us the series?

'Three, eight, one, four.'

'Four, one, eight, three.'

I'm so sick of not being there at the end of big matches.

'Six, two, nine, seven, one.'

'One, seven, nine, two, six.'

Sent off in the World Cup semi-final.

'Seven, one, eight, four, six, two.'

'Two, six, four, eight, one, seven.'

Injured against France for the Grand Slam match.

'Walk in tandem gait towards that wall, please. The back of your lead foot against the toes of your rear foot.'

Did my hamstring in Melbourne four years ago.

'That's fine, thank you. You've done that in good time. Do you have a headache?'

'No.'

My head's a little sore from the impact, but no more.

'Do you have any dizziness?'

'No.'

If this was a club game, would I be off?

'Do you have any pressure in your head?'

'No.'

But it's not. It's my last game ever.

'Do you feel nauseated or do you feel like vomiting?'

'No.'

I've got the rest of my life to recover.

'Do you have any blurred vision?'

'No.'

I promised myself that I'd be there at the end today.

'Does the light or noise worry you?'

'No.'

And that I'd lift the trophy on the pitch, bloody and sweaty and muddy.

'Do you feel as though you're slowing down?'

'No.'

I've heard no more huge cheers. It must still be 15–12.

'Do you feel like you're in a fog?'

'No.'

Let me back out there.

'Do you feel unwell?'

'No.'

Let me back out there NOW.

'That's fine, Sam. You've passed the assessment and can return to the pitch.'

Back up to pitchside, as fast as I can. It is 15–12 to them, I was right. I look at the clock. I've been down there with the medics seven minutes, give or take.

I come back on at the next break in play.

Faz and Rhys take down Dagg between them and win the scrum. Even a put-in at this stage feels as huge as a penalty. The scrum's good. Very good. Our front row are massive, forcing theirs down and giving us the kick. I'm fired up, slapping their heads as they come up.

Too far out for Faz to go for goal. Maro takes it into a ruck. I clear out Faumuina. The All Blacks are on the wrong side, stopping Rhys from getting the ball, and he's furious, slapping Crockett and appealing to Poite.

Penalty. Three minutes left. Here we go again.

Faz lines it up, of course. The man could tap dance in a minefield. Cool as you like, he brings us back to all square, 15–15.

Two minutes left. Titanic match. Titanic series. Not over yet.

Beauden Barrett kicks off. Liam and Read jump for it. The ball comes off Liam to Ken, who's right next to him and slightly in front. Instinctively, Ken catches the ball – he's had a split second to react – and in the same movement he opens his hands and drops it, knowing that he's offside.

Too late. Poite blows. Penalty to New Zealand.

Penalty to New Zealand with two minutes left. I can't believe it. This is just so textbook New Zealand it's ridiculous: to win it right at the death after everything we've thrown at them, after we've been toe-to-toe for the best part of four hours and you can hardly fit a fag-paper between us.

I yell at the boys to watch for a quick tap. There's nothing we can do if they take the shot at the posts, but to lose because we've switched off and they tap and go would be something I'd never get over.

Poite seems to be consulting with the TMO. I go over and ask him to check Read's challenge in the air, to see whether he'd fouled Liam when they were both jumping for the ball. It's an air shot at this stage, but I've got nothing to lose. If you don't spend your chips with two minutes to go and the series in the balance, when do you spend them?

I take a mouthful of this liquid we have to stop cramp, as I've been cramping like crazy these last few minutes. We're not supposed to swallow the liquid, but just squirt it in, slosh it around inside our mouths and spit it out again: it works on the receptors inside the mouth.

Read comes over to where I'm standing, next to Poite. We bump fists lightly, recognition that we're both at the heart of something very special.

'Wow,' he says. 'This is rugby.'

They're showing the whole incident on the big screen. There's so much to unpick there at pretty much every stage, almost frame by frame. Was Read in front of Beauden Barrett, the kicker, at kick-off? Was Read's challenge in the air on Liam legal? That is, could he reasonably have hoped to get to the ball himself? Did Read get a hand to the ball himself, which might mean an All Blacks knock-on? Did the ball come forwards off Liam, or was it lateral?

There are four or five possible decisions here, and some of them might not just cancel out the All Blacks' advantage but swing it the other way. If Read is deemed offside from the restart, for example, we'll have a scrum on halfway. Imagine that they drop that scrum and we have a kick to win it. Not just that, but we have a kicker to win it too: Elliot, with his monster boot.

The only thing that is totally beyond doubt is that Ken was in front of Liam when he played the ball. So he's definitely offside. But was it deliberate, or accidental? This is what Poite's discussing with the other officials.

The whole thing hinges on this. Deliberate offside is a penalty, but accidental offside's only a scrum.

The relevant sections of the laws are 11.6 and 11.7.

11.6 ACCIDENTAL OFFSIDE

(a) When an offside player cannot avoid being touched by the ball or by a team-mate carrying it, the player is accidentally offside. If the player's team gains no advantage from this, play continues. If the player's team gains an advantage, a scrum is formed with the opposing team throwing in the ball.

   (b) When a player hands the ball to a team-mate in front of the first player, the receiver is offside. Unless the receiver is considered to be intentionally offside (in which case a penalty kick is awarded), the receiver is accidentally offside and a scrum is formed with the opposing team throwing in the ball.

11.7 OFFSIDE AFTER A KNOCK-ON

When a player knocks on and an offside team-mate next plays the ball, the offside player is liable to sanction if playing the ball prevented an opponent from gaining an advantage. Sanction: Penalty kick.

The laws are slightly contradictory, not to mention rather ambiguous. What does 'play the ball' mean? How about 'cannot avoid being touched by the ball?' No professional player, used to catching hundreds of balls in training every week, can decide in a fraction of a second *not* to catch a ball that comes to them; to do so would be to override an instinct drilled so deep within them as to be more or less muscle memory by now. This was why the Scots were so furious to lose the World Cup quarter-final two years ago to Australia: an offside that was deemed deliberate but that they said was accidental.

All this, I think – I *hope* – is playing in the minds of the officials. No one wants any series settled on such a contentious decision, let alone a series which has been as momentous as this one has.

There's about half a minute of Poite discussing things with the TMO before he comes over to Read and me.

'We have a deal,' he says. 'We have a deal about the offside 16.' It's maybe not the best word to use, 'deal' – it implies some sort of agreement cooked up – but I think he means 'decision' and, in the heat of the moment speaking in a language that's not his own, he picked slightly the wrong word. 'He did not deliberately play the ball, OK? It was an accidental offside.'

Read's not happy. 'No, no, no.'

'It was an accidental offside,' Poite repeats. 'So scrum for black.'

'Romain,' Read says. 'Romain.'

But Poite's made his mind up. I intertwine my fingers together so the boys can see. Scrum. Get in position and pack down before he can change his mind again.

Just over a minute to hold them out.

The scrum wheels. Read loses control at the base. Rhys steals it and legs it downfield. He passes inside to Toby, who can't quite hang onto it. Knock on. Another All Black scrum. The hooter goes. Next time the ball goes dead it's over, but if any team can win from here it's the All Blacks; if any team has the skill, the patience and the balls to work it for two, three, four minutes at the end of 80 lung-busting minutes, it's them. It's never over against these guys until it's over. They always play right to the end, and you can never let up because you can be sure they won't.

Ardie Savea comes through. I hold him up. They're in our 22. Cruden flips it over the top to Jordie Barrett, who slips Elliot and goes for the corner. Liam hauls him down, and CJ and Faz bundle him towards touch. Perenara has it, a couple of metres out. Men all over him, driving him up and back and out. The flag is up.

The final whistle goes. I grab a 500 ml bottle of electrolytes and neck the lot, ready for extra-time – and then I look up and see that everyone's shaking hands.

It's over.

It's over?

I honestly thought we'd have extra-time, as though this was the knockout stage of a World Cup. If the series hinges on it, why not do so? But apparently a draw's a draw, unless it's been agreed otherwise beforehand.

It feels a weird anti-climax. Read's still talking to Poite. No one really knows what to do. The interviewers grab us for quick pieces to camera.

'Wow,' I say. The crowd are quiet, waiting for me to continue, and then they realise that I don't really know what else to say and they burst into applause. By the time the applause subsides, I can just about formulate some words. 'What a Test match. It's difficult. It's all geared to winning. It's better than losing, I guess.'

'I feel pretty hollow, to be honest,' Read says. 'I'll look back on it in the future with a bit more pride.'

I find my dad, Ben and some of our mates in the crowd. They've been yelling for me, but I couldn't hear them above the din. I give them a hug. We're not a touchy-feely family, but it's an incredibly emotional moment.

I'm called back for the presentation. In 2013, I shared the trophy lift with Alun Wyn. Now I share it with Read. We take the trophy between us, each with one hand on one handle, and raise it together. I tug it towards me, playfully. He laughs and tugs it back, neither of us quite ready to quit fighting for it even now.

I remember the vow I made to myself four years ago: to be here, as skipper, on the pitch, lifting this trophy, the one time my body didn't give out on me. And it's come true, sort of. It's come true, except I never envisaged that Kieran Read would be on the other end of the trophy. Mind you, if you asked him, I bet he never thought that I'd be on the other side of any trophy he was holding, so it all evens out.

'Would you have gone to extra-time?' I ask him.

'Absolutely.'

I wish we could have pulled rank. Perhaps at this level, with everyone out on their feet, it would have been dangerous to go another 20 minutes, so I'd have played a golden point: first team to score wins, simple as that. Try, penalty, drop goal, doesn't matter. As a spectacle, a climax, that would have been unbelievable.

Kaino walks past us. 'Shall we get the boys in?' he asks. 'All of us together?'

It's a great idea. We call everyone in and get them to mix, so we're not just sitting in our own teams but in among the opposition and vice versa. There's Rhys with his arm around Dagg, Kaino with his hands on Toby's shoulders, Ken with Ardie Savea, red and black mingling as one – a great image, an iconic image, of two teams that took each other from pillar to post and back again. Forty-six guys who gave everything, won nothing but came away with something special. They couldn't separate us over three matches, and they can't separate us now.

No one likes a draw, not really. But if you'd told me when we left Heathrow that, with only six weeks' preparation and having been ahead for only three minutes across three entire Tests, we'd have shared the series, would I have taken that?

On one level, no. Professional rugby's about winning. We won in Australia in 2013; we didn't win here. For that alone, Australia would be the one I'd take if you offered me only one of those series. But in playing terms, the 2017 series was a greater achievement, no doubt about it. The Australia team we beat was a good one. The All Blacks team we drew with was a great one. Add to that the quality of the non-Test opposition, the toughness of the schedule and the relentlessness of being in a country where rugby feels as important as a religion, none of which applied in Australia, and the differences between the two are clear.

We could have won, no matter how unlikely people thought it. We could have won, and part of me will always be annoyed that we didn't. We certainly could have done more. It was the pinnacle of everyone's career, and it lasted six weeks. For six weeks you'd have thought it possible to dedicate yourself totally to the cause, wouldn't you? For six weeks, you could leave no stone unturned when it came to making sure you performed at your absolute peak: eat right, sleep right, stay off the booze as it's bad for recovery from inflammation, stay away from the blue light of mobile phones, and so on.

But I reckon only 20 per cent of the boys could honestly say they did that for the duration of those six weeks, which, given that we took 41 players, means around eight players. Just over half a starting XV, just over a third of a match-day 23. When you think how close we came, would it have made a difference – would it have made the crucial difference – if everybody had done that? Very possibly. And it's no accident that some of the ones who *did* apply themselves properly were among the best performers on that tour: Maro and Alun Wyn in the second row, Johnny and Faz at 10 and 12.

It would have been nice to have had a neat and tidy ending, but sometimes you don't get them, in sport as in life. A drawn series is very rare – only once before in Lions history has it happened, and that was back in 1955. In the modern era, it's unique. As Gats says, draws aren't the worst thing in the world; they create scenes like that joint team photo, which expresses the joy of rugby better than anything else I've seen. That photo, and the result which led to it, will forever set the 2017 Lions apart. That's not a bad way to be remembered. Not a bad way at all.

LEADERSHIP 7: PEOPLE

A rugby team is a collective, but everyone within that collective is an individual. Those individuals can be, and usually are, very different from each other. Each person in the squad has his own strengths and weaknesses, his own hopes and fears, his own areas of confidence and insecurity. Being able to get the best out of people is key to being a leader. Some people need a kick up the arse every now and then; others need an arm round the shoulder. Knowing which is which is crucial. Get it wrong and you can do more harm than good.

But you can only do this if you know people. You don't have to be everyone's best mate or remember the name of their wife's hairdresser's second cousin, but you do need to know what's important in their lives. Warren Gatland was very hot on this, both for Wales and the Lions. Tell us what's going on at home, he'd always say. If things are good at home they'll be good here, in training camp or on the pitch; if they're not, then they won't be.

No one can keep their home and work lives inseparable, not forever. If your wife needs a scan, tell us. If your kids are ill, tell us. If your parents need help, tell us. Family always comes first. Sometimes leadership is about giving people time rather than taking it from them. And people remember this. Say you lose them for a day or two, even for a week or two. Further down the line, they'll remember the kindness and sympathy you showed and will work even harder for you.

Ben Youngs pulled out of the 2017 Lions tour because his sister-in-law, Tiffany, was suffering from cancer. Tiffany's husband Tom, Ben's brother, had been a Lion himself in 2013, and knew how all-consuming and demanding a Lions tour is. There's no point having someone on tour whose mind is understandably elsewhere. Besides, family is life. Rugby's just a game.

As captain, I did my best to be as available and inclusive as possible. If I came into lunch and saw three tables full of people, I'd go and sit at the one where I knew fewest of those people well.

There were three reasons for this. First, it let me get to know them better, which in turn allowed me to help them more, or to go to management and say, 'X is struggling a bit with this.' Second, it meant they'd be more likely to come to me with a problem or a suggestion. And finally, it stopped any perception that I might think myself better than other people, or be part of a clique with my own favourites.

Of course you get on better with some people than with others – that's just human nature – but as captain I couldn't be seen to be hanging around with just the Blues guys when I was playing for Wales, or just the Welsh lads when I was with the Lions. This was also why, with a few exceptions such as the 2017 tour, I always preferred to share a room rather than use the captain's preroga-tive and have one on my own.

That determination to be seen as neutral and unbiased extended to my relationship with Gats and the management staff. I was captain of the team, which meant my loyalty was to the play-ers first and foremost. I never wanted preferential treatment as a captain; I never wanted not to have to fight for my place, or to know things that other players didn't, or be seen in even the slightest way as representing the management rather than the players.

I got on well with the coaches, of course, but my loyalty was rightly always with the players. So I never sat in on selection committee meetings or the like, even though Gats told me I could if I wanted to (and part of me did really want to, as it would have been fascinating. Sometimes on the Lions videos there's a clip of the coaches discussing a player who's obviously not named for their own privacy, and you're thinking, *Ooh, I wonder who that is they're talking about!*).

I also did my best to empower players and give them roles. Any leader who wants to take everything on themselves and not trust anybody else to do anything is harming the team and making it all about himself, in which case he shouldn't be leader in the first place.

This worked both off and on the pitch. Off the pitch – and especially for the Lions, where you're on tour for longer and boys start off not knowing each other that well – I'd set up various committees to get people involved and give them ownership of various aspects of the tour. Laundry, ents (find out what to do and where to go in the places we'd stay), fines for various misdemeanours (this was always the easiest one to select; just give it to the front row, as no one argues with them), and rooming.

Rooming I always thought was an important part of leadership. Some people liked to keep mixing players up, so they'd get to know new blokes every time they moved hotel and therefore avoid the danger of cliques. I disagreed. Sharing a room is quite an intimate and personal thing, especially in the tense times before a match, and you need someone you trust and feel comfortable with. It can be stressful if you're sharing with someone you don't feel that easy with, or who has different habits to you: watching TV late when you're trying to sleep, or bouncing around the room at dawn when you want a lie-in.

So I always liked to see guys in with people they knew well. If you want to get to know someone better, there are plenty of places to do it – at training, on the bus, in the team room – and then, as often happened, you can ask to share with each other next time round; but, crucially, because you want to rather than because you've been told to.

On the pitch, I was never the sole leader; I always had several others around me. For Wales, there were guys like Alun Wyn, Gethin and Jamie Roberts; for the Lions, Johnny Sexton, Jamie Heaslip and Geoff Parling. In the case of the Lions, men like Sexton and Heaslip in particular were very vocal, which suited me fine. Heaslip was so motivational in the dressing-room, so loud and talkative, that he did much of that stuff for me. Did I need to repeat what he'd said just because I was captain? No.

A leader who trusts in his own position is happy for others to speak up. Before the second Lions Test in South Africa in 1997, who was standing in the middle of the huddle before the match, geeing up the Lions? It wasn't Martin Johnson, the skipper; it was Scott Gibbs, who was player of the series. As long as the team gets the right message, it doesn't matter who says it.

As captain, I actually had relatively few jobs on the pitch. It started with the coin toss, where I'd always follow the advice of my old mate and mentor Martyn Williams: 'Tails for Wales never fails.' If I won the toss, I'd have to choose whether to take the kick-off or ends. At Cardiff with the roof closed it was easy, as there was no wind to consider, so I'd always take the kick-off; we kick, they catch, we belt the carrier, they clear their lines, we get an attacking lineout 35 metres out. But in other stadia I'd consult with the kickers and the coaches first.

Then, during the game, most decisions I had to make were also in some way dependent on other people. Penalty 45 metres out: go for the posts or the corner? That depends on how the kicker's feeling. Free-kick: run it or take the scrum? Again, that depends on how the scrum's going that match, as well as how well we're attacking and they're defending, so the pack leader and scrum-half's opinions might come into play.

The one area where the captain can exert a significant influence by himself is in communicating with the referee, as only the captain can speak to the referee without the referee first speaking to him. And the relationship between referee and captain is one of the crucial ones in the game. Rugby, especially at international level, is a complex sport where judgement calls can be both very marginal and very important. Being on good terms with the referee isn't an option; it's a necessity.

I got a lot of attention over the years for the way in which I dealt with referees and the rapport I enjoyed with them, to the extent that sometimes I was seen almost as the Referee Whisperer, capable of making them do what I wanted with some sort of Jedi mind tricks. I wish! If I did have a secret, and I didn't, it was just by applying the same principles to them as I did to my own team-mates, and indeed to everyone in life. It was basic people skills, nothing more.

Think back to school. In almost every class there was a kid who never shut up and was always badgering the teacher. It doesn't take long for the teacher – and everyone else, for that matter – to treat whatever that kid says as just white noise. So too with captains and referees. Some captains are always chuntering away, but referees just tune them out.

I asked Nigel Owens about this once – he trains full-time with the WRU so he's often around with the national team – and he confirmed it. 'We know what we're looking for,' he said. H H Almond, who took charge of the first ever rugby international between England and Scotland in 1871, once said, 'when an umpire is in doubt, I think he is justified in deciding against the side which makes most noise. They are probably in the wrong.'

I always tried to be well mannered, not just with referees but everyone, and careful not to waste time and energy arguing over every point. It's what every aspiring lawyer is taught on the very first day at law school: the quiet voice can often be the most persuasive one. Less is more.

Romain Poite always said, 'you can speak to me twice a half: three times if I'm having a bad game.' I was like, 'ah mate, that's perfect.' I liked this for two reasons. First, it gave me defined parameters to work with, and in doing so forced me to assess what was worth bringing up and what wasn't. I didn't want to spend my chips highlighting something irrelevant if ten minutes later there was something important which I couldn't bring up as I'd already used my slots. Second, Poite's acceptance that he could and did have bad games was refreshingly honest. Everyone has a bad game from time to time: players, referees, coaches. Everyone's human.

Other refs would say, 'Don't speak to me when the clock's on.' That was fine too, because that also helped me pick my moments. The time to ask wasn't when the referee had just made a big decision; I'd still be emotional and any doubts would still be in his mind. At the next break in play, when everybody had cooled down a bit, that was the time to ask.

In the second Lions Test in 2013, I wanted to know why Craig Joubert kept penalising Mako Vunipola in the scrums, but I waited not just until there was a break in play but also for my opposite number Stephen Moore to finish speaking with him. It gave me a few extra seconds to calm myself and showed respect not just for the referee but the game too.

And, as always, I asked a question rather than made a statement. Asking a question of the referee did two things. It made him give me an answer, which meant we had dialogue, and it also implicitly accepted his authority. Imagine I was pinged for offside when I was convinced I was onside. I could either remonstrate – 'No way was I offside there!' – or ask, 'Why was I offside there?' No prizes for guessing which one would have been more likely to get me a favourable response.

My relationship with the referee wasn't a one-time static thing. At club and international level I came across the same officials again and again, so the better I got to know them, the better I could play when they were officiating. With Nigel, even though of course he couldn't referee me at international level, I was always chatting to him and picking his brains, not just because he's an interesting bloke but also because I never knew which bits of information or advice I might be able to tuck away and use one day.

This ongoing relationship also stemmed from one simple fact about referees, and indeed life: I couldn't change the past. No ref was going to alter a decision he'd already made; it would weaken his authority too much, and that would be no good either for him or for the game itself. But I *could* influence the present and the future.

In terms of influencing the present: say the opposition had scored a try and the ref had gone upstairs to check that the ball was grounded properly. While that was happening, I could ask him if he could get them also to check a possible blocking or offside earlier in the move. He might not have acted like he'd heard, but as often than not he'd ask anyway. Refs don't mind having their attention drawn to things; what they mind is looking like they're giving in to players.

In terms of influencing the future: say my opposite number wasn't rolling away at the breakdown. I could use a lull in play to ask the ref to keep a lookout for this. Perhaps in 10 or 20 minutes' time he'd ping that player for precisely the offence I'd mentioned. Would he have done so otherwise? Maybe. Maybe not. But it never hurt to ask.

A wider version of this is the kind of meetings that coaches (and sometimes captains) have with referees the evening before a match, when they raise concerns – tacklers going for a kicker's standing leg, for example – which they want policed. Both sides in any match do this, and they have every right to. If you don't, you can be sure that your opposition will.

Sometimes, especially since I played 7 and was consistently contesting the breakdown, the whistle would go against me personally. I would never protest when this happened, but I *would* ask for clarity. Against Scotland in 2013, when Joubert was once again the ref, he penalised me at a turnover. The rule was that you had to release the player you'd tackled just for a split second before getting on your feet and jackalling over him. 'Was that for unclear release?' I asked. He said yes. 'Do I need to release sooner?' I asked. Again he said yes. This way, I knew how much he'd let me get away with, and he knew I'd taken his instructions on board.

Nigel Owens once pinged me for the same offence. As I got up, I said, 'Are you sure, Nige?' 'You're quick,' he said, 'but not that quick.' With a smile, I countered, 'I'm pretty quick, mind.' Nothing cutting or nasty. Nothing strident or overtly critical. But he admitted later that the comment acted as a marker, as I'd hoped it would, and he made a point of taking a closer look at the next breakdown.

As a leader, therefore, it's all about people, whether those people are referees, team-mates or coaches. Treat them with respect and listen to what they want, and not only will you keep them happy, but you'll also improve the performance of your team, which is – or should be – your ultimate aim.

EPILOGUE

July 2017. When I ran out at Eden Park for the third Test against the All Blacks, I was convinced this was my last match ever, at any level. Looking back, I was only ever at 70 per cent in that series.

But of course I still have a contract with the WRU and the Blues, and now I'm back from New Zealand and away from all the insane pressure of the Lions goldfish bowl, I start to think that maybe I was too hasty. There are still plenty of things left in the game for me. And I'm only 28. That's way too young to retire.

The physios give me a scan.

'Your body's in pieces,' they say. 'Pretty much everywhere we look there's a problem.' Few of the problems are that big in themselves, but as with the way I felt after the 2015 quarter-final against South Africa, it's the accumulation of them all that really gets you down.

'Is there a technical term for all this?' I ask.

'Yes.'

'What is it?'

'The technical term is: "You're screwed."'

I drop all my Lions kit off at the Tenovus Cancer Care charity shop in Rhiwbina. It raises £3,000 in two hours, which in terms of what they need is a drop in the ocean, but which is at least better than nothing and also helps to raise their profile a tiny bit and get them in the news.

A couple of people go on social media to accuse me of 'an act of self-promotion'. Sometimes you feel as though you just can't win.

August. The usual lay-off period after a season is four weeks. I'm so exhausted and beaten up by the end of the Lions tour that these four weeks go in a flash. Normally, by the end of this period, I'm gasping to get going again. Not now. I'm still in physical pain, and mentally I'm nowhere near the right place to put my nose back to the grindstone. I ring Derwyn and tell him I need another four weeks. He says he'll sort it with the WRU and the Blues.

I go for a run. Actually, it's not so much a run as a trot. And it's awful. I feel old, slow and shit. For the first time ever, I don't want to do pre-season training; me of all people, who's always been Mr Preseason. At this rate I won't be up to speed in time for the autumn internationals in November. Maybe I should just sack off them completely and aim for the start of the Six Nations another two or three months down the line.

What's really strange, though, is the change in my mindset. Even during the worst of my injuries, I've always tried to keep being positive. Sure, there've been plenty of times I've hated the stress – hence all the mid-match retirements in my head! – but I've never been so … apathetic, I guess. I'm loving not having to train, and the thought of playing doesn't excite or scare me, it just makes me feel down. When you're used to either absolutely loving or absolutely hating your sport, and sometimes going from one to the other in the blink of an eye, not really caring is a very unusual and very difficult thing to deal with.

I'm not depressed, but I'm definitely mentally affected by it all. This uncertainty is so not me. I've always been used to being decisive and positive, but right now I feel neither. And at the heart of it is the same feeling I had during the calls for me to be dropped during the 2012–13 season; if you define yourself as being an athlete, and all of a sudden you're not that athlete anymore, then who are you?

Rach and I have been together a decade. She's never seen me like this, and she doesn't really know what to do. How could she? I don't even know what to do. I do know that if this goes on much longer it will start to put a strain on our relationship. My mindset will change, I'm sure of it. It will change. It has to.

September. I come back to training with the Blues. After eight weeks off, I'll need at least three weeks before I touch a ball again – up until then it's just physical preparation – and another week beyond that before I'm ready to play again, but suddenly Ellis Jenkins is injured and we may need me to cover for him in a fortnight's time.

This is not what I need. I need to be taking it slowly, to be focusing on my body so I can get my mind back to where I need it to be. But I also know how patient the Blues have been with me over the years, and I want to help them any way I can.

I do some gentle pad drills. I jog into a tackle pad, shoulder first, at 50 per cent effort, tops. I bend down to place the ball … and feel my neck go again. A stinger, just like I've had so often before, but from the gentlest of contacts. I stop the session immediately.

Injury #23.

On the video (all training is filmed), it looks so innocuous. Inside, though, my mind's churning. *This is ridiculous, how often this is happening.*

Nick Williams has a calf problem and is out of the next match against Leinster. We might need you on the bench as cover, the coaches tell me. The physios are having none of it. You can't play, they tell me. You categorically cannot play.

I'm grateful to them, because something is very wrong here. I can't sit in the car for more than 15 minutes or so before I get a burning sensation between my shoulder blades that is so bad I need to pull over and flex my neck. Of all the parts of your body to mess with, the neck is not one. Things have never been this bad before. Right now I can hardly live a normal life, let alone play rugby.

My head's not right because my body's not right. They're not separate things. They're interlinked. My head's right when I'm playing well. I play well when I'm physically fit. If I'm not physically fit, my head won't be right. A simple circle of never-ending cause and effect.

The solution is simple. Get my body right and the rest will follow. Getting my body right will require a change of approach. It'll need surgery.

* * *

I talk to Gats, and I talk to the WRU. I need two operations, one on my neck and the other on my knee, and between the two of them they'll keep me out for the season. A complete break from the game until the end of the season. I offer to go unpaid, which makes Derwyn put his head in his hands. A player unilaterally volunteering to forgo his salary: it's every agent's worst nightmare. No, the WRU say, there's no question of you being unpaid. But I think they appreciate the gesture anyway.

I go in for the neck op. They're going to shave the bottom of one vertebra and the top of another just to help that gap where the nerve comes up, because it's when the nerve is compressed that I get the stingers.

They ask me to sign a disclaimer form – it says that, since they're operating so close to the spinal cord, I accept there's a 1 in 1,000 chance of paralysis. I know it's a very remote chance, that these numbers always seem theoretical and that all surgery carries some kind of risk, but it does make it seem just that little bit more real. I think of Owen, in a wheelchair for life. He's doing great now – fundraising for others who've suffered sporting injuries, and he's in a relationship with his carer – but the spectre of what he's been through is never far away at times like this.

Normally I look forward to operations, if only for the feeling of dozing off under anaesthetic and then for the morphine afterwards: that sensation of being on Cloud Nine and not giving a toss. But today I'm really nervous. Before I go into theatre, I post a photo with Anna on Instagram. It's the first time I've ever been nervous for an op, because it's the first one I've had since becoming a dad.

It's not just about me anymore. It's about Anna and any brothers and sisters who come along. I see the ex-pros walking around with these big, swollen knees and they can't do anything. I don't want that to be me. I want to go down to west Wales in 10 or 15 years' time and be an active dad. I want to be an active granddad in 30 years' time.

The first thing I see when I walk in is this massive head clamp.

'What the hell is *that*?' I say, trying to make a joke of it.

'Well,' the surgeon says, 'after we put you under we turn you 180 degrees onto your front, and then we put that clamp on so that your head can't move, not even a millimetre.'

'OK,' I say. 'In that case you'd better put me under right now, because I'm about 20 seconds from freaking out and legging it into the streets of Cardiff wearing nothing but this paper gown.'

I remember the breathing techniques Andy used to teach me before matches – green energy in, red energy out – and I use them now while waiting for the anaesthetic to kick in.

Next thing I know, I'm waking up in a hospital bed in floods of tears.

'How are you feeling?' the nurse asks.

'My neck is absolute agony and I feel really sick.'

'That's to be expected. That's what operations are like.'

Well, I think, this is my seventh, and none of the others have been remotely like this. If someone told me that I'd feel like this for the rest of my life, I'd rather die, I honestly would, and I'm someone who's always been afraid of death. It's like that line about seasickness going through two stages: when you think you're going to die, and when you're afraid that you won't.

'Can I have a bowl, please?' I ask.

They bring one. I projectile vomit twice in ten minutes.

'F*** rugby,' I say, loud and angry, when I'm sure my stomach's empty and all I have left is dry retching.

November. Walking the dog in Rhiwbina. A couple of builders working on a house down the road see me, give the thumbs-up and shout, 'Living the dream, Sam!' I laugh and wave at them, but inside I'm thinking, *If only you knew.* If only you knew that in a few minutes' time I'll turn the corner and walk past the local rugby club, and I'll watch them playing and see the enjoyment they take from the game, and I'll try to remember when I last felt something that pure and uncomplicated about the sport that's defined me for so long.

December. Now the operation on my knee. It's got 1.5 cm of lateral movement, which is ridiculous. The ligament's basically just hanging off. If you push my kneecap, it glides. Even with all the strapping I put on it, I'm only one serious collision away from blowing it properly; one big tackle, one big hit while jackalling. At my age, that's a year out of the game. In this case, prevention is definitely better than cure.

I go under the knife. The surgeon puts a synthetic medial ligament in, nice and tight and as good as new.

My body's patched up now. No more excuses.

January 2018. New Year, and new me – or rather old me, young and hungry and competitive. It's like a switch has been flicked. I'm lifting as much in the gym as I ever have, and I'm feeling great. My body's getting better, and as it does I can feel my mind following suit: body leading the mind, as it does so often in this most brutal of sports.

I hear the whispers on the grapevine: Warby's done, he's gone, he's never going to be the same player again. And when I hear them, I feel the old response bubbling up in me: *You're wrong, and I'm going to prove it to you.*

I set out some personal goals I still want to achieve. I want to win the Six Nations player-of-the-tournament award, and be nominated for World Player of the Year, neither of which I've ever managed and both of which I feel I should have achieved. I want to captain Wales to the 2019 World Cup, which would be my third as skipper.

March. I give an interview to *The Times*, and my positivity's reflected in the quote. 'I will play again. I can say that 100 per cent.' I'm watching games. I'm visualising myself playing those games. I want to be back out there.

The Blues ring me. We know you're on sabbatical, they say, but our injury list is mounting. If we need you to cover – and we'll only ask you in case of dire emergency – could you do it?

I go for a run. It's only 3 km, but I have to stop three times. My knees are agony; they feel like bone is rubbing directly on bone, with all the cartilage having been worn away.

I ask Rach whether she feels pain like this. Of course I don't, she says.

I phone Ben and tell him what's happened. You're stupid, he says. You're in rehab for your knee. You can't just run on it without any prep; you have to build yourself back up into it.

That's true, I know it is. But what's also true is that a normal 29-year-old man can put on his trainers and go for a run – a very short run – without having to think about it.

My body leads my mind. And if my body's not up to it, my mind won't be either. This doesn't break me, but it definitely bumps me. Deep inside my head, a little voice says two words.

Strike one.

April. I begin training with Foxy, Rhys and Scott Baldwin. It's a nice little training group, and I'm soon in good shape, good enough to think I'd be ready to play tomorrow. But deep down, I know I'm kidding myself. The training is just conditioning, with straight-line running and no actual rugby, and even then I have some pain in my neck when doing overhead presses in the gym and in my knees when I run. I could deal with muscle soreness, but this is different. This is pain deep within the joints.

May. At the end of the training block, Prav gives me an advanced knee rehab session. He has me bounding left and right, changing direction again and again.

'Be more explosive!' he says.

I try, but I can't move any quicker.

'Snappier! I want to see you snappier!'

The pain comes jabbing through both knees like white-hot needles. I have to stop. That was agony, and yet I know what he was asking me to do wasn't – shouldn't have been – anything out of the ordinary.

Strike two.

Monday, 9 July. I start pre-season with the Blues. My knees can just about stand up to it as long as the physios give me pain-killing jabs directly into them. I kid myself that this is normal, that they'll somehow get better in time. As long as I can still function on them, that's OK, right?

Tuesday, 10 July. We're in a huddle after finishing our Blues training session. Some of the senior players and coaches are talking. I'm not really listening. I'm a bystander, looking at the grass, and I'm thinking *This is it. That session was so hard, what with all the changing of direction. My knees are so sore. Imagine two people now flying into the side of those knees. I can't do it. It's 14 months to the World Cup. I'm never going to make that.*

I pick up Anna from nursery. Back home, in the garden, she asks me to go on the trampoline with her. Bouncing with Daddy: it's one of her favourite things. I crawl onto the trampoline. She thinks I'm playing around, being silly. I'm not. My knees won't let me do anything else.

'Stand up, Daddy,' she says.

I try. I can't do it. I'm on all fours trying to push myself upright, and it's just too painful. I can't even kid myself it's DOMS (delayed onset muscle soreness), as I've had that for 15 years and I know exactly what it feels like. This isn't it. This is very far from it.

'Daddy.' Anna's voice is more impatient now. 'Stand up, Daddy.'

I grit my teeth and make a huge effort.

'For God's sake!' I shout, not because Anna's asking me to stand up but because my knees are so painful. My voice is loud and deep and angry, and it scares Anna so much she bursts into tears. I'm on my feet now, but with the shifting surface of the trampoline below me my balance is all over the place, and it honestly feels as though my knees are going to dislocate if I stand here a moment longer, let alone if I try to bounce.

Strike three.

I sink to my knees again, cuddle Anna and tell her I'm sorry. Then I take her inside. I crawl off the trampoline and gingerly walk across the garden through the back door while she walks alongside me. Normally I'd grab her and take her upstairs with her laughing and me tickling her, but now I have to get her to go ahead of me while I go up the stairs on all fours.

While Anna plays, I sit and think, just turning it all over in my head.

I don't want to be that player who's just hanging on, holding a pad. If I can't get to the heights I want to, the heights I'm used to, there's no point in keeping on; and I can't get back to that level, I know I can't. My body just can't cope with the volume of running any more. They might say I only have to train twice a week and ice my knees for three hours a night, but that in itself would be the end. I'm not Ledley King, who was so good that he could turn up every Saturday without training and still play top-quality football. I'm not blessed with flair, and you can't play rugby without the training anyway, it's not that kind of game. If I'm not physical then that's a lot of my game gone. All in or all out. That's how I've always played. No half measures. Go hard or go home.

Rach comes home. I tell her what's happened, and that I've had enough. She's surprised, both because I've seemed so much better these past few months, and also because she's heard it all before.

'I love this sport,' I say, 'but I hate how it makes me feel sometimes. And I know you've heard me say that time and time again. Everyone hears that, but no one listens. No one properly listens.'

She looks at me, and she knows. She doesn't try to talk me out of it. She knows as well as I do.

I'm done.

I send Derwyn a text message.

Hey mate,
Just wanted to give you a heads up. I'm not calling because I won't really be able to speak and I've got a little emotional talking to Rach about it.

    I've been back two days, and all the same feelings I had last year are straight back again. It's confirmed to me I really don't want to continue as a player. I genuinely was looking forward to coming back and playing, but after doing some rugby, and contact preparation etc the thought of playing really doesn't appeal and I guess the only way I can say it is I can't keep doing this to my body and I have no motivation to train. I've been the best pro at the ground the last two days' training and for my whole career and I love getting myself in shape, but the thought of playing and future injury worries me. I'm trying to play with Anna since I got home and I'm struggling to even be on the trampoline and pick her up. My knee is f*****, my back is f***** and I've had a tits full.

I'm going to sleep on it, and I'm finding it hard to talk to Rach, because it's almost that realisation, and it's so hard to speak about it because I feel I'm letting so many people down. I'll give you a bell tomorrow but just wanted to plant the seed.

Cheers mate.

Wednesday, 11 June. I've slept on it, and my mind's still as resolute as it was yesterday. I ring Derwyn and tell him.

We work out a plan: who do we need to speak to? As few people as possible, at this stage. We don't want the information coming out piecemeal before we've had the chance to sit down with the people who really need to know and explained the decision to them.

My family apart, all of whom are totally supportive – 'I knew the night you rang from Wellington that it was over,' Mum says, 'there was just something in your voice. You spoke too strongly, too passionately' – the first names on that list are obviously the WRU and the Blues, both of whom I'm contracted to.

And, even though right now he's at home in New Zealand with his family, I have to tell Gats, because he's put so much faith in me for pretty much my entire career. I ring him. He tells me I've done the right thing: family comes first, just like he's always said.

Friday, 13 July. I go to see the WRU at the Principality. It's the hardest meeting I've ever done. I can't shake the feeling of deep, deep guilt. They've been so good to me: arranging my operations with top consultants, taking me up and down to London, paying me as usual and never once pressuring me to come back.

And in return, I've told them I'm quitting. I'm afraid they'll think of me as some journeyman chancer who never had the slightest intention of coming back, but just took the money and had a laugh. It couldn't be further from the truth, of course, but maybe that's what I'd think if I were them, and I wouldn't blame them for a moment.

I start to explain myself. It's taking every ounce of energy I have not to break down right here in the meeting room.

'Sam, let me stop you there.' It's Julie Paterson, head of operations. 'The only reason I wanted you to come in here today was to look you in the eye and see that you really mean it. And you do, that's as clear as day. That's all I wanted to know. You've got nothing to apologise for. Absolutely nothing.'

She stands up, comes round the table and gives me a hug.

Through the windows I can see the pitch and the stands behind: the best stadium in the world, the place where I've had some of the best memories of my life. I'm turning my back on all that. I'll never again run out through the flames and the dry ice, never again see the three tiers banking up to the heavens all around me, never again stand on the pitch with 'Land of My Fathers' crashing all around me.

It breaks my heart, but I know it's the right thing to do.

Tuesday, 17 July. We decide to make the announcement at midday tomorrow.

I ring my two best mates in rugby, Lyds and George, and tell them. I also tell the medical teams at the WRU and the Blues, because without them I'd have been doing this five years ago.

I tell the Blues I'm not coming in tomorrow. Personal reasons, I say, and leave it at that. Less is more.

Wednesday, 18 July. I'm at Heathrow, on the way to a family wedding in Italy.

It goes on Instagram at midday: a picture of me walking out at the Millennium, together with a message I wrote myself.

Unfortunately, after a long period of rest and rehabilitation the decision to retire from rugby has been made with my health and wellbeing as a priority as my body is unable to give me back what I had hoped for on my return to training.

I cannot thank the Welsh Rugby Union and Cardiff Blues enough, who have gone beyond the call of duty in providing the support I received to help me get back on the field, for which I will be forever grateful.

Since I first played aged 10 at Llanishen Fach Primary School, then Whitchurch High School and Rhiwbina Juniors RFC, I always dreamed of playing for my hometown club the Cardiff Blues, Wales and the British and Irish Lions. To look back on my career, I'm extremely proud of what I managed to achieve. There are so many people who helped me along the way from schoolteachers, coaches, friends and family. I thank you so much for supporting my dreams and aspirations. I hope they too can take some pride from my career.

I would like to make special mention of Warren Gatland. Without the faith he had in me and his unwavering support I would never have had the career I was able to pursue.

Countless people work behind the scenes in professional rugby but I would like to thank the fantastic medical teams at both WRU and Cardiff Blues who have looked after me throughout my career.

To my amazing wife Rachel and my close family and friends who have endured the emotional rollercoaster of playing professional rugby, I am so lucky to have such a fantastic support network and loving family to help me get through all the testing times.

Lastly, to all the many fans, with whom I've shared some fantastic memories, from the bottom of my heart, thank you so much for all your support. From providing a random hug in a supermarket, or simply offering words of support and encouragement, to hearing a cheer after my name was announced at the national stadium, you are what makes playing professional rugby so special and such a privilege. It's been an absolute pleasure to represent you all and an honour I'll sorely miss.

As one chapter finishes, another begins, which I'll enter with the same level of passion and determination as the last. Thanks.

The flight is at 1 pm. I'm going through security when all of a sudden my phone starts going mental. Some of the other passengers in the queue obviously see it come up on their news feeds when they're looking at their phones, and they're looking at me like they can't quite believe it. There's a massive TV screen in the departure lounge and suddenly I'm on it. I knew it was going to be news, but I had no idea it was going to be this much news. I feel a little like I've died!

Rach takes Anna into the children's soft-play section. They won't let me in as I'm wearing flip-flops, and you need to be wearing socks. So while they're in there I scroll through the stuff on my phone. There are hundreds of messages and notifications, so much so that my Twitter feed can't load them all up. I've had big news days – announced as Lions captain, important World Cup wins, Grand Slams – but this is another level.

The messages I do get to read are so heartfelt and complimentary that I can't believe it. In the nicest possible way I had no idea that people, not necessarily players but fans, had that much of a nice opinion of me, thought that much of me. I really had no idea. It's so unexpected and touching that I feel myself getting emotional and starting to tear up, so I put the phone away before I give some paper a headline tomorrow. **WARBURTON, BROKEN BY RETIREMENT, HAS EMOTIONAL MELTDOWN IN DEPARTURE LOUNGE.**

And that's it. No more Sam Warburton, rugby player. Just Sam Kennedy-Warburton: father, husband, son, brother.

It's weird. It's good. Rugby's what I did. It was never who I was.

March 2019. I've been retired nine months now, and I can honestly say I've loved every minute of it. I heard somewhere that two-thirds of rugby players get depressed when they finish playing. Sometimes I felt depressed when I *was* playing! It might sound ungrateful, given all the things that rugby gave me, but it's true. Not clinically depressed, perhaps, but certainly ground down at times.

Retirement feels really good. I know it is the best thing for my body and for me. Every day that's passed, I've woken up and known I've made the right decision. Even when Wales were going for the Grand Slam earlier this year, I never wanted to be out there with them. I wondered if I would, wondered if at the moment of their supreme triumph I'd feel a sense of bitterness and jealousy, but I genuinely didn't. I was just delighted, absolutely delighted, for them all.

I haven't had an ounce of regret. It feels like a massive weight off my shoulders. I can carry Anna up and down the stairs fine, I can play with her on the trampoline. I know I'm not going to spend tomorrow morning in an operating theatre dosed to the eyeballs on morphine, or tomorrow afternoon getting stitched up under the stands with concussion.

All the scrutiny you get from the press, all the rehabilitation from injuries, the pain of playing, the mental strain of repeatedly getting yourself up for big games, the pressure you put on yourself, people not respecting your time, the emotional side of things that your family goes through, your parents getting stressed out about stuff – I don't miss any of those things. Not one bit. Not one tiny bit.

I do miss one thing. I miss those moments in the dressing-room before or after a match, preparing for or recovering from the supreme effort, summoning up the sinews as I looked into my team-mates' eyes and knew they wouldn't let me down, or slumped on a bench after a titanic victory, too shattered to move but with every fibre of my being suffused with the deliciousness of knowing we did it.

* * *

I'm not famous, and I'd never want to be. David Beckham's famous. Will Smith's famous. That's the kind of fame that must skew your life, when everybody thinks they know you and has an opinion about you long before they ever meet you. I'm locally well recognised, certainly in Wales and at rugby grounds around the world, but that's pretty much it (and even then people mistake me for George North, which he finds devastating as he thinks he's much better-looking than me). Rach and I went to New York not long after my retirement, and for an entire week there no one gave me a second glance. It was glorious.

I'm busy doing lots of stuff. Writing this book, obviously. Writing a column for *The Times*. Doing commentary and analysis for the BBC at the Six Nations, BT Sport for club matches and ITV for the World Cup. Being an ambassador for the WRU. Keeping up work with my sponsors. Busy enough not to be bored, but not so busy as to never have a moment to myself. It's perfect. I keep fit and have lost several kilos. I'm still training like stink, but not eating as much. I was never supposed to be as big as I was.

What I like about rugby is that it doesn't come with all the ridiculous hoopla that football seems to. I do my own social media, because that makes what I put up real, and people appreciate that. I don't have a whole team posting things as me and ensuring that everything's refined and on message to within an inch of its bland life. When I go somewhere for work, I don't need an entourage around me or a driver who'll chew my ear off for three hours. I like to drive myself: get in the car, chuck on talkSPORT, stop for a coffee and a pee when I want, and then claim the miles back at the other end!

As for the longer-term future, who knows? I know what I don't want to do, and that's be a head coach. When I see the pressure that's been heaped on Gats over the years, the unforgiving nature of the media and the public, I wouldn't put myself through that, and I certainly wouldn't put my family through that. I wouldn't leave my kids open to struggling in school, or my folks to being abused in the street, because everyone was slagging me off.

But there are lots of other roles within rugby that are less in the public eye. I'd like to do some mentoring work one-on-one with people. I'd like to help coach strength and conditioning, which were always among my favourite parts of the game. Perhaps when Bobby hangs up his coaching boots, the Bobby Cup could become the Warby Cup! I'd like to help get the Blues to a European title in whatever capacity suits them and me best.

And I'd love one day to be Lions manager; not the coach but the manager, who acts as a figurehead and conduit off the field, who helps pull all the players and staff together, and who's always available to help out someone who for whatever reason is struggling a bit. To be Lions manager would be a great, great honour.

Sometimes I look back and think to myself: did I have it easy? Did I play so many games for Wales and the Lions, was I captain so many times, only because the coach liked me? On one level, perhaps, it doesn't matter. Just like every other player, I had the career I had, no more and no less.

But I'd be lying if I said that even now I keep all the negative thoughts away. I never questioned my ability while growing up, but when you're at the top and everyone's queuing up to take pot shots at you – sections of the press, social media, even some of your own team-mates – then of course some of it starts to filter through.

Almost no player is lucky enough to finish their career with no regrets at all, with nothing left undone. I'm no exception. There are things I'd love to have done. I'd love to have won another trophy for the Blues. I'd love to have reached 100 caps. I'd love to have skippered Wales in a third World Cup and skippered a third Lions tour. But none of them were to be. You can drive yourself crazy with 'what ifs?', and they do you no good. Better, and easier, just to be grateful for what I did have.

Whenever you've been around a while and achieved some things in the game, people will always try to rank you. In the immediate aftermath of my retirement, many people were kind enough to call me a 'great player' (a description to which Stuart Barnes, unsurprisingly, took exception), and whenever pundits and writers choose their all-time Wales XVs, I'm in there more often than not.

Whether or not I was a great player is for others to decide, not me. What I will say is that I don't see myself in the very top drawer of those who've played the game. I was at the top of my career for only six or seven years, whereas men like Brian O'Driscoll and Paul O'Connell were at the top of theirs for much, much longer. I won 74 caps for Wales; Richie McCaw won exactly twice that number, 148, for New Zealand.

Clearly there's more to a career than just longevity. But, given the intense levels of competition at the top of the game, those who can stay there not just for a handful of years but for knocking on a decade and a half are obviously a cut above the rest, both physically and mentally.

I was never one of those, and I can live with that.

I still live in Rhiwbina. We've got one more bedroom than we did, but that's as flash as I get. My brother lives across the road, literally; he bought my previous house off me. My entire family live within half a mile. I love it here. Why would I move? This is where I live. This is my house.

And if you come to that house, there's only one item of rugby-related memorabilia on show: my first Test Lions 7 jersey, framed. Other than that, nothing. I don't even have a rugby ball in the house. I'd make a terrible *Through the Keyhole* guest.

One day I'll build a little room, more for my own memories than anything else. I've already earmarked the first seven things that will be going in there:

- That Lions Test jersey I just mentioned.
- My Grogg, that's for sure, as if you've got a Grogg then you've made it in Wales! Groggs are small clay figurines of people, and of course the more distinctive your features the more the makers have got to get their teeth into. When I was first asked to do one back in 2010, the guy taking pictures of me said – and I knew exactly what was coming – 'No offence, but you've got a fantastic face for a Grogg.' I'm sure there was a compliment in there somewhere. They made one of me in the strip of every professional team I played for, which meant the Blues, Wales and (later) the Lions. They also said they'd do one of me in an amateur

jersey, so which one would I choose? I could have gone for Glamorgan Wanderers, whom I played for while still at the Blues academy, or Rhiwbina, but I chose Whitchurch, as that was where so much of my formative rugby education and love for the game was forged. They made two of me in a Whitchurch strip, and I gave one to my PE teacher Gwyn Morris along with the Lions shirt I wore in the first half in Brisbane in 2013. He got rather emotional, though maybe that was just the thought of having to see my ugly mug on a Grogg every day.

- The luxury watches we received on the Lions tours. Breitling made the 2013 edition and Bremont the 2017 one. Both have got my name, cap number and Lions emblem engraved on them, and unlike replica shirts they're not on sale to the public; they're purely for those who play for the Lions, and you have to earn them the hard way. (Some of the 'geographical six' asked for them in 2017, which as you can imagine didn't go down well.) I guess they're sort of the Lions version of the Superbowl ring.

- The traditional Maori knife I picked up from the ground when we were given a Maori welcome in New Zealand.

- The boots I was wearing when Alain Rolland sent me off in the 2011 semi-final, because that single incident, more than any other in my career, made me as a person. I had to go from boy to man, and very fast. I wasn't proud of the red card, but I was proud of the way I responded to it.

- From the same tournament, the greenstone man of the match award I won against South Africa, not just because it's very rare for someone on the losing side to win man of the match, but also because that was the game in which I really announced myself as a proper world-class 7, up there with the big boys.

- A frame of both captain's jerseys from the Wellington Test in 2017, mine and Kieran Read's (which was also his 99th cap).

It won't be a big room; there won't be space for much more than one or two people. It'll be just somewhere I can go now and then to look back and remember that, for all the things I never managed, there was an awful lot that I did.

The memories I have are very special, Kipling's twin impostors of triumph and disaster alike. I'm very lucky to have them, and I'm very proud to have shared them with you as fully and frankly as I could – to have shown you my open side.

APPENDIX A

THE FUTURE OF THE GAME

Rugby is at a crossroads. The issue of player safety is, quite rightly, at the very top of the agenda of everybody who cares about the game. It's been almost a quarter of a century since the game went professional, and in that time certain aspects have changed almost out of all recognition. In particular, players are bigger, faster and stronger not just than ever before but perhaps than their amateur predecessors could ever have dreamed of.

I did think of calling this book *Too Big, Too Fast, Too Strong*, not just because many people see rugby this way but also because when you're a professional, that's almost what you're encouraged to aspire to. If you're too big, too fast and too strong, after all, you'll be a better player than your opposite number.

But first things first. Rugby is a contact sport; it always has been, and hopefully it always will be. If you don't like that, there are plenty of other sports out there you can go and watch. Rugby's a contact sport because there's a demand for it, both from players and spectators. The physical contest and the alpha

369

male desire to impose supremacy on an opponent are not just woven deep within our society, but deep within our DNA, deep within our own cells.

If you were an alien beamed down to the Principality on match day, with the hits and the cheering, what would you think of humanity? Whatever it was, it wouldn't be inaccurate. Incomplete, perhaps – you'd obviously get a different impression if you landed in a library – but not inaccurate. It goes back to ancient times, when crowds of ancient Romans would fill the Coliseum to watch gladiators kill each other.

Sport, and particularly sports like rugby, are our way of replicating and perpetuating that desire while couching it in enough rules to ensure that the violence remains within acceptable bounds. The single most important reason I played was for that confrontation, that physical battle.

I needed that, and I make no apologies for it. In the stands at the Principality or on the pitch, you can shout 'Smash him!' and no one bats an eyelid. Try that in a nightclub or on the street, and you'll end up in the back of a police van. Better to do it on a pitch, with a referee and TV cameras and spectators, and then shake hands afterwards.

So any discussion about the future of rugby must take this into account: that the sport exists for a reason, and that reason tells us things about ourselves that we might not want to hear. But we do need to change things. The bottom line is that the game is evolving faster, much faster, than the human body. Players do much more strength and conditioning work than they ever did, honing muscles and cardiovascular systems to a fine peak, but underneath it all the skeleton is still the skeleton.

I'm living proof of this, forced to retire before the age of 30 because my body just couldn't take it anymore. You could leave me out for scrap and the tinkers would take me away. I've got a pin in my left shoulder, another pin in my right shoulder, a plate in my jaw and another in my eye socket.

And I'm one of the lucky ones. People are dying on rugby pitches. In the seven months between May and December 2018, there were five deaths recorded during a match or as a direct result of playing rugby. Three of them were in France. Nicolas Chauvin, an 18-year-old academy player at Stade Français, broke his neck in a two-man tackle. Adrien Descrulhes, 17, was found dead of a brain haemorrhage the morning after suffering a concussion playing in an Under-18s match for Billom. Louis Fajfrowski, 21, suffered a heart attack after being hit in a tackle while playing for Aurillac. The other two were in Canada, where 18-year-old Brodie McCarthy died after a collision while playing for his school in Prince Edward Island, and South Africa, where 31-year-old Kyle Barnes died of a head injury in a club match.

At Stade they call their young players *espoirs*, 'hopefuls'. Nicolas Chauvin never got a chance to make good on that hope. It's up to us all to ensure that those who come after him do get that chance. Rugby's just a game. It's not worth dying for. And if something isn't done soon, then a professional player will die during a game, in front of the TV cameras, and only then will people throw up their hands and demand that steps must be taken. It will be reaction rather than anticipation, cure rather than prevention.

Head injuries are, of course, usually the most problematic and serious. World Rugby is quite rightly very hot on its concussion protocols, which are light years better than they were when I first came onto the international scene. They are also trialling reducing the height of the tackle to below nipple level, which may help. But ball-carriers will still lower their own heads when charging, and tacklers will still get bounced off teak-hard upper bodies and suffer head whiplash that way. You can't stop people running into each other or putting their heads on the wrong side. You can't eliminate the risks entirely.

What you *can* do is reduce them, most obviously in reducing the amount of time players spend on the pitch and the nature of the work they do while they're out there. If I were World Rugby supremo with *carte blanche* to do what I like, I'd do the following, in four main areas: contracts, time limits, substitutes, and jackal protection.

Contracts. In order to guard game time, centrally contract all regular international players. The international game is rugby's showpiece and provides the bulk of the sport's revenue. This isn't football, where at least the more successful clubs have followings as large and rabid as national teams. The Rugby World Cup is a lot nearer football's World Cup than the Heineken Cup is to the Champions League. In any club–country debate, country has to come first.

Time limits. A limit of 25 games per player per season. I know it's a vicious circle with the need for enough games to pay wages and the like, but there has to be a limit somewhere. There would have to be discussion around this, of course. What constitutes a 'game' in this context? A minimum period of time on the pitch? Being part of the starting XV or the match-day 23? Given that 25 games of 80 minutes equals exactly 2,000 minutes, perhaps this could be set as the limit instead, obliging teams to work out how best to use up these minutes.

Full-contact training limited to 10 minutes per week. This would be just in the professional game (not at junior, amateur or semi-pro levels where the hits aren't as big), and wouldn't include semi-contact, such as mauling practice, or work with pads and tackle bags: just full-on bone-on-bone contact work. Allowing players to recover between matches in this regard is paramount. I didn't like contact in training, not because I didn't like tackling – I *loved* tackling – but I wanted to protect myself so I could be as physical as possible on a weekend.

A minimum of 12 weeks between the last game of a season and taking full contact again, and within that a minimum period of no organised training whatsoever. Ideally this would be six weeks totally off, followed by six weeks of no-contact training, but a three-stage approach (five weeks totally off, five weeks pre-season and two weeks semi-contact) may be more achievable given the current calendar.

Substitutes. Reduce the number of subs allowed. At the moment, more than half the team can be replaced, which means that some players – especially tight-five forwards – can bulk up to the max in the knowledge that they'll only have to play around 50 minutes rather than 80. Add to this the mismatch in energy when fresh blokes who've just come on are clattering into those who've been playing the whole match, and the potential for injury is doubly clear.

In one area, the problem perpetuates itself: for safety reasons you need a full complement of front-row subs, but these guys are of course the biggest units who can cause the most damage. But beyond that, perhaps have one more forward sub and two backs, making a total of six rather than eight. It would be nice to go back to the old amateur ethos of only bringing on a sub for injury, but let's be honest, in the professional game that's never going to happen.

Protection of the jackal. Referees need to start enforcing Law 15.7, which states that 'a player must bind onto a teammate or an opposition player. The bind must precede or be simultaneous with contact.' This would reduce the momentum of the clear-out players and therefore their ability to seriously injure the jackal.

Nor is it enough just to look at the professional game in isolation. One of the best things about rugby is the wide base of the pyramid, a long way below the narrow, rarefied heights of Premiership and international rugby: the clubs, the schools, the teachers, the volunteers. If we lose these, then we lose the whole game.

And we are in danger of losing them. Maybe not yet, and maybe not by much, but even the smallest backslide can quickly snowball into something greater. If parents are too worried about the prospect of serious injury to let their children play rugby, then we lose two generations to the game: the current schoolboy one and the next adult one.

And parents *are* worried, even – especially – the ones who know the game well. Former England full-back Nick

Abendanon said: 'I don't think I will push [my son] to play rugby when he gets older.' Mick Cleary of the *Daily Telegraph* wrote in December 2018 that 'for the first time in 50 years of playing and reporting on the game, I have reservations about encouraging kids to take up the sport.' Even Will Greenwood, World Cup winner and in his own words 'one of the biggest advocates for the sport that you are ever likely to meet', said that 'if my kids told me they did not want to play anymore, a (very) small part of me would probably be relieved.'

I understand where they're coming from, especially now that I'm a dad myself. But I want to balance this with all the things rugby has given me. If I were looking to mould a top-class 7 from schoolboy level, I'd be looking as much at his character as his physique. Yes, he'd have to be an athlete, big and strong and adept enough to learn technical stuff like lineout work and jackalling; but more than that, he'd have to be someone of substance.

He'd have to want to learn, to improve, to listen to coaches. He'd have to be tough; tough enough not just to handle the knocks and disappointments but to come back for more, to be the kind of person who might fall eight times but will rise nine. These aren't just rugby qualities; they're life qualities. Rugby helps us build character and promotes good qualities; sportsmanship, teamwork, respect, fitness, camaraderie, self-esteem and so on. It's imperative that we keep these qualities, that we don't throw the baby out with the bathwater.

The international game. Rugby has a great opportunity to expand both east and west, to Japan and the USA. Both countries have the money and infrastructure to come on leaps and bounds in the next decade or so, perhaps not to the stage where they'll be showing the All Blacks a clean pair of heels, but certainly no more than a level or so down from that. A World Cup semi-final between Japan and the USA? Easily possible.

Talking of the World Cup, it's not so long ago that the idea of Japan hosting the tournament seemed unlikely, if not outright laughable. It would be great for the game if the USA got to host the World Cup sooner rather than later. Perhaps Japan 2019 will be a catalyst for something like this.

Six Nations. The most obvious problem is Italy. Their white-wash in the 2019 tournament was their fourth in succession, a losing streak that actually goes back a little further: 22 losses on the bounce, with their last win coming against Scotland in 2015. Having one team out of six that is more or less a guaranteed win reduces the intensity of a tournament in which every other match is contested like a fast and ferocious derby.

In 2019, Wales put out more or less a second team against Italy. In terms of player protection and game management you can't blame them, but the ethos of the Six Nations has always been that your best team takes the field. That's why I was so thrilled to get my first Six Nations call-up in 2010. Anything that dilutes this is not fair on the tournament, and it's not fair on Italy. They're getting better, there's no doubt about that. The problem is, so is everyone else.

But what to do about it? I'd like to see relegation to and promotion from the second tier, but this is unlikely for one good reason: the Six Nations would collapse if England ever got relegated. The TV numbers would plummet and the sponsors would scarper. I can see that Georgia and Romania in particular want it to happen, as they're the best of the rest, but they also know that money talks (and that, rightly or wrongly, most rugby fans would prefer a weekend in Rome to one in Tbilisi or Bucharest).

The club game. Some of the issues that apply to the international game also apply to the club game, and in fact I'd like to see more integration between both categories north and south; a superseason, if you like, with the Six Nations and Championship played at the same time, and top-level club rugby north and south the same.

Promotion and relegation will also dog any attempts to reform the club game, but that's no reason not to try. I'd love to see a 20-team Home Nations league, with 10 clubs from England and 10 from Ireland, Scotland and Wales combined; but who'd agree to start off in Division 2? And what would happen if all the teams from one of the smaller countries ended up in Division 2? Their attendance and viewing figures would go through the floor.

The Lions. Last, but absolutely by no means least, are the Lions. The 2021 tour to South Africa will only have eight games rather than the 10 we had in New Zealand and Australia. To my mind, this is exactly right, providing that the Lions get two whole weeks together (the first in Britain or Ireland, the second in the host country) before they take to the field for the matches proper.

In both 2013 and 2017, we could have happily scrapped both the first match and the midweek match before the first Test without making any difference. Four matches before the first Test mean most of the squad will get two starts and everyone will get two games; keeping the midweek match between the first and second Tests means that everyone who plays in the final Test will have played no more than 10 days before, ensuring they're match sharp.

I don't know much about the finances and politics of it, but from a playing perspective the Lions is the most special thing you'll do in your international career. Don't believe it? I did a sponsorship event with Lawrence Dallaglio, one of only a dozen men to have been part of a winning Lions squad and a winning World Cup squad. When it came to the Q&A, someone asked about exactly this: 'Lawrence, you've won the World Cup, and you've won a Lions series. Which was better?'

Ooh, I thought. *That's a good question. I really want to know the answer.*

Lawrence didn't even have to think about it.

'The Lions,' he said. 'Hands down, the Lions.'

The Lions must continue, no matter what direction world rugby takes from the crossroads at which it currently stands. The Lions are the embodiment of most, if not all, of rugby's best values, and these are too precious to lose.

APPENDIX B

MY BEST WELSH XV

I played 74 games for Wales and was lucky enough to line up alongside and against some fabulous players in that time. These are the best of them.

First, the best Wales XV, plus replacements, of my time in the red jersey. I reckon this lot would be a match for pretty much anybody.

15 Leigh Halfpenny. Pence had everything. He ran great lines at pace, he tackled well and his handling was sublime. But most of all, his kicking was almost flawless. Having a kicker like Pence is invaluable for any captain, as it means you have a banker three points every time the opposition concede a penalty within range. In fact, some teams we played against changed their tactics purely because of Pence, choosing to compete less at the breakdown for fear of being pinged. There were games we won almost exclusively because of him.

14 George North. He's been around so long that it's easy to forget that he's still relatively young. To score a brace of tries aged 18 against South Africa, light up the World Cup aged 19 and score the greatest individual try in Lions history aged 21 all show what a prodigious talent he was, and remains. Pace, power, hunger – he's got the lot.

13 Jonathan Davies. The greatest players do it for the Lions above all, and Foxy's been immense on two Lions tours. He was player of the series in 2017 and wasn't that far off it four years before (when he played two of the three Tests out of position). Even at aged 16, word was getting round about him, a kid from the Scarlets who was just smashing every fitness test going. You don't realise how good he is until you play with him.

12 Jamie Roberts. For a man who started top-flight rugby in the back three, Jamie didn't just adjust fast to playing 12; for a while he was the best 12 in the world. Most players slow down slightly when they take the ball into contact – it's a human reaction. Jamie was the only person I played with who actually ran harder into contact. His handling and footballing skills were very underrated, and his reading of the game as defensive captain was excellent. He'd be a very good defensive coach if the medical career doesn't work out ...

11 Shane Williams. Even in training, aged 33, he was putting other wingers to shame. Shane was one of those rare players who always looked as though he'd do something whenever he had the ball, who always had the crowd rising. He was lightning quick, his sidestep was absurdly good, and when he popped up as first receiver he could conjure play from nothing. And in a game that can often seem all about size, he was proof that the little guy can still rule the roost.

10 Stephen Jones. A century of caps is testament to his skill and longevity. He was the ultimate cool head and pair of safe hands, experienced and calm, and understood the game so well (as is evident from the way he's gone about his coaching job at the Scarlets). He was also deceptively strong. Once while playing in a Blues–Scarlets match, I had the ball and saw that he was flanked by a couple of props. I'll run over the weedy 10, I thought. He hit me damn hard! I thought twice before trying that again.

9 Mike Phillips. As with Jamie, there were times when he was the world's best in his position. Insanely competitive, he played more like a ninth forward at times, keeping opposition back rows honest all afternoon long. A big-match player – the greater the occasion, the better he performed. Yes, he could be arrogant, but that's what you want in a scrum-half. He was also one of the funniest guys I ever played with, sometimes walking hunched over and explaining to anyone who asked that he had a bad back from carrying this team for so long.

1 Gethin Jenkins (c). One of the easiest picks in this team. Gethin could do everything: scrummage, tackle, carry, breakdown work. One of the fiercest competitors out there, and also one of the canniest. His reading of the game was so good that it was like having a coach on the pitch with you.

2 Matthew Rees. The competition for the hooker berth on a Lions tour is always really fierce, so for Matthew to play all three Tests and start two of them in 2009 shows you how good he was. He was big enough to play back row, and a warrior from the old school, the kind of guy who never took a backward step and just got on with things.

3 Adam Jones. Super strong at the height of his powers. A consistently dominant force in the scrum, which – given that the tighthead prop is the cornerstone of any scrum – made him such an important part of our successes. His going off so early in the 2011 semi had at least as much of an influence on the game as my red card.

4 Bradley Davies. One of the most amazing athletes I ever played with. He could offload from the back of his hand, drop goals from the halfway line and sidestep like a Fijian – all of this encased in the body of an international lock. His lineout understanding was world class. Were it not for his atrocious luck with injuries, and the fact that he peaked between Lions tours, he'd have been a starting Lion for sure.

5 Alun Wyn Jones. As much of a shoe-in as Gethin. Big and durable – way more than 100 caps in a very attritional position – he hardly ever has a bad game, and as a captain he's been inspirational to players and fans alike. A pretty much unanimous choice for 2019 Six Nations Player of the Tournament.

6 Dan Lydiate. The uniqueness and effectiveness of his chop tackle made him one of the few players to single-handedly revolutionise defensive systems. A freak, in the nicest possible way. Coaches would come specially to watch his gym sessions as he lifted such huge weights.

7 Martyn Williams. The hardest decision in this XV, because Justin Tipuric is such a talented player, but Martyn just shades the openside berth. He won man of the match so often when Wales were doing well that sometimes the award seemed almost routine. People forget quite how good he was. My childhood hero, and every bit as great a bloke as he was a player.

8 Toby Faletau. The best all-round player I played with. He has so much ability and talent, more I think than he even appreciates. He doesn't know how good he is. He can do everything. He was almost uncoachable, because he was always in the right place at the right time. He could easily have played 13 at international level.

If I had to pick one example of his absurd talent, it was against England in 2015. We had a scrum that England disrupted, shoving us backwards and wheeling at the same time. Toby dipped his hand between the second row's feet, plucked the ball out against the drive and the wheel, beat three players and offloaded to Rhys Webb for the try – in other words, turned an overload into an overlap. I can't think of another player in world rugby, not even Read or Parisse, who could have done that.

Subs:

16 Richard Hibbard. One of the most physical players out there. He was always on the physio's bench as he constantly wrecked himself, flying into every contact like a rocket. A great bloke to have around any team.

17 Paul James. A strong scrummager, an experienced operator and a tackler almost as good as Lyds on his day.

18 Samson Lee. So strong that he could hold a scrum even aged 20. An Achilles injury halted his progress for a while, but he's back now and his ball-carrying has vastly improved.

19 Luke Charteris. Best defensive lineout player I ever played with – his long octopus arms could control a lineout maul on their own. A superfit guy with a great engine; when you consider that at 6 ft 10 it's a long way down to the deck and up again, and when you consider that hitting 40 rucks a game is good going, his figure of 57 against Samoa in the 2011 World Cup is very impressive.

20 Justin Tipuric. The fittest and most skilful forward of my time. Like Toby, he could have played 13 at international level, and there's not an outside centre who wouldn't have been proud of his running line and dummy to set up Cuthie for the winning try against England in 2013. A lot more physical than people give him credit for, too.

21 Rhys Webb. An old-school 9: cheeky, gobby, sniping, and will sell you a dummy every game. Lost years to injuries, so would have been even better than he is. If this was just about hair and skin, he'd be first name on the teamsheet.

22 Liam Williams. Can cover all positions in the back three. Great all-round ability, and an annoyingly good natural sportsman; you just have to watch him playing tennis or golf to see how good his hand-eye co-ordination is.

23 James Hook. Deservedly popular with the fans; always used to get a huge cheer when he came off the bench. A mercurial talent who could play 10, 12, 13 and 15. As a 10 he tended towards the Carlos Spencer end of things sometimes, where Gats often preferred a more conservative Jonny Wilkinson style.

APPENDIX C

MY BEST INTERNATIONAL XV

And second, the best international XV I played against. These guys are pretty useful too, to say the least …

15 Israel Folau (Australia). If I were a club's director of rugby and solely selecting someone on rugby grounds, I'd choose him. He can do almost anything.

14 Bryan Habana (South Africa). Everyone knows how quick he was. But he was also solid and very strong.

13 Brian O'Driscoll (Ireland). His highlights reel, longer than almost anybody else's, shows his skill and flair. It doesn't show what a great jackaller he was; in all seriousness, better than quite a few international 7s.

12 Ma'a Nonu (New Zealand). Began as a one-dimensional bosh merchant. Ended as the most complete inside centre in world rugby.

11 Julian Savea (New Zealand). The bus: big, quick, strong and with a great step. His try-scoring record at international level is phenomenal.

10 Jonny Wilkinson (England). One of my all-time heroes. I wanted to be like him – I saw how hard he trained, and I modelled myself on that.

9 Will Genia (Australia). Always played really well against us, which was very annoying. A good bloke, too; texted me commiserations after my injury in Melbourne with the Lions, a gesture I really appreciated.

1 Andrew Sheridan (England). A monster at loosehead with powerlifting stats out of this world.

2 Bismarck du Plessis (South Africa). Massive both in stature and around the park.

3 Carl Hayman (New Zealand). The world's best tighthead for a while.

4 Paul O'Connell (Ireland) (c). A leader and Lions legend, as tough as they come.

5 Sam Whitelock (New Zealand). One of the best lineout operators and a mainstay of his team.

6 Jerome Kaino (New Zealand). An almost perfect 6. Great at all the unseen work, legal and illegal, and would bend in half any player who ran at him.

7 David Pocock (Australia). The single hardest player I ever faced. Not so much a thorn in the side of opposition teams as a human JCB.

8 Kieran Read (New Zealand). Like Toby, could have played 13 at international level. Did everything round the park.

Subs:

16 Guilhem Guirado (France). Old-school French hooker: skilful and hard.

17 Cian Healy (Ireland). A devastating athlete.

18 Tadhg Furlong (Ireland). A massive man who will only get better.

19 Maro Itoje (England). So talented and influential for one so young.

20 Richie McCaw (New Zealand). Even the name is enough.

21 Aaron Smith (New Zealand). Whip-quick pass and a great communicator.

22 Dan Carter (New Zealand). Magisterial in his pomp.

23 Stuart Hogg (Scotland). Like Shane Williams, but with muscle.